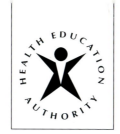

health
update

sexual health

[2ND EDITION]

1997

ISBN 0 7521 0697 X

1st edition, 1994
2nd edition, 1997

Health Education Authority
Hamilton House
Mabledon Place
London WC1H 9TX

Compiled by:
Rose Hunt (Research consultant)
Joanna Goodrich (HEA)
Mary Sayers (HEA)
Henrietta Lang (Research consultant)

Additional contributors:
Paige Sinkler (HEA)
Hilary Whent (HEA)

Series Project Manager:
Paige Sinkler (HEA)

Acknowledgements
We are grateful to Antony Morgan and other colleagues at the Health Education
Authority, the Public Health Laboratory Service (AIDS Centre) Communicable
Diseases Surveillance Centre, the Family Planning Association, the Department
of Health, and the Bureau of Hygiene and Tropical Diseases and Mark Fitzgerald
of the British Federation Against Sexually Transmitted Diseases, for their
comments on earlier drafts and editions of this *Health Update*.

Contents

Summary facts

SEXUAL BEHAVIOUR
- The median age of first sexual intercourse for today's 16–24-year-olds is 17 years of age. (p.7) Over half of all 16–19-year-olds report having had sexual intercourse. (p.12)

- Only 10% of respondents aged 16–74 in one national survey thought that someone like them had a 'very high' or 'quite high' risk of infection from HIV. (p.10)

- In another survey, 32% of men and 19% of women said they would use a condom if they had sex with a new partner. (p.11)

CONCEPTIONS
- There were 801 600 recorded conceptions in England and Wales in 1994. (p.13)

- It is estimated that between one-third and one-half of conceptions are unintended. (p.13)

- Among those under 16 years of age, 52.8% of conceptions led to abortion in 1994. (p.13)

CONTRACEPTION
- Use of oral contraceptives has declined from 28% of 18–44-year-old women in 1983 to 25% in 1993, while the proportion of women whose partners used the condom rose from 13% to 17% between 1986 and 1993, with the largest increase among 18–19-year-olds. (p.17)

- A national survey found that 86% of 16–19-year-old men, and 91% of 16–19-year-old women reported using at least one method of contraception at first intercourse, mainly the condom or the pill. (p.20)

- One study found that 70% of women requesting an abortion in a 1990 study said they would have used emergency contraception but did not know how to obtain it; 30% were unaware of the option. (p.22)

ABORTION
- In 1995 153 135 abortions were performed on women resident in England and Wales. (p.24) After an increase in abortion rates in the 1980s, rates have declined. In 1995 these dropped 2.2% from 1994. (p.25)

- High teenage abortion rates in the UK compared to other European countries have been attributed in part to poor access to family planning services. (p.25)

- Since July 1995, RU486 (mifepristone) has been available for use in medical abortion between 13 and 20 weeks gestation. (p.27)

AIDS AND HIV
- By the end of June 1996, a cumulative total of 27 088 HIV reports had been recorded in the UK. In 1995, there were 2684 new reports of HIV in the UK. (p.30)

- Men who have sex with men form the largest proportion of new AIDS cases each year. In 1995, 63.1% of all new cases were in this category. (p.30)

- New reports of HIV infection among heterosexuals, though low, continue to increase. The proportion of new infections contracted through heterosexual intercourse increased from 8.3% in 1989 to 19.6% in 1995. (p.31)

- The 1996 Day Report estimated that almost 49% of adults living with HIV may not have been identified. (p.35)

OTHER SEXUALLY TRANSMITTED DISEASES
- Sexually transmitted diseases other than HIV are a major cause of ill health and can have long-term consequences including infertility, ectopic pregnancy and genital cancers. (p.38)

- The *Health of the Nation* target for gonorrhoea has been surpassed. In 1995, there were 12 359 new cases in GUM clinics in England, 5% above the total for 1994. (p.39)

- The number of cases of chlamydia rose by over 15% between 1993 and 1995 to 39 289, the highest since 1989. (p.40)

SEX EDUCATION IN SCHOOLS
- A number of studies suggest that sex and AIDS education do not promote earlier or increased sexual activity in young people. On the contrary, they may lead to an increased uptake of safer sexual practices. (p.43)

- Sixty-one per cent of primary and 76% of secondary schools have a sex education policy. (p.44)

- Four-fifths of parents interviewed in an HEA study in the UK said they think sex education in schools should include information on how to use a condom. (p.45)

Introduction

The World Health Organization has defined sexual health as 'the integration of the physical, emotional, intellectual and social aspects of sexual being, in ways that are enriching and that enhance personality, communication and love'.

WHO has defined three elements which should inform discussions of sexuality and health:

- the capacity to enjoy and express sexuality without guilt or shame in fulfilling, emotional relationships

- the capacity to control fertility

- freedom from disorders which compromise health, and sexual or reproductive function.[1]

HIV/AIDS and sexual health have been identified as a key area in the Government's White Paper, *The Health of the Nation: a Strategy for Health in England*.[2] 'Good personal and sexual relationships can actively promote health and well-being. On the other hand, sexual activity can sometimes lead to unwanted pregnancies, ill-health or disease'.

Thus, the two main targets are:

- To reduce the incidence of gonorrhoea by at least 20% by 1995 (baseline, 1990), as an indicator of HIV/AIDS trends.

- To reduce by at least 50% the rate of conceptions amongst the under-16s by the year 2000 (baseline, 1989).

While acknowledging that sexual health covers a broader range of issues than is covered here, this *Health Update*, like others in the series, reviews those areas for which quantitative data are available.

Data relevant to sexual health and public health are not always comprehensive or reliable, and compiling this publication has highlighted the need for improvements in data collection and presentation. The data come from a wide variety of sources and are published at varying intervals. However, the intention of this *Health Update* is to be as up to date as possible.

Comments and suggestions for improvement are always welcome.

Sexual behaviour

INTRODUCTION

Surveys of sexual behaviour in the general population provide key information for the understanding of the epidemiology of HIV and other sexually transmitted diseases. Information on sexual behaviour also informs the design of prevention strategies and sex education initiatives.

Sexual behaviour of relevance to public health policy are those practices which put individuals at risk of contracting a sexually transmitted disease or unintentional pregnancy, or which inform policymakers about the context in which potentially 'risky' sexual practices are undertaken.

Collecting information on people's sexual behaviour is not straightforward; there may be unwillingness on the part of interviewees or respondents to admit to some activities, including anal and oral sex, and certain sections of the population may be less willing to answer questions on sex.[1] There have been very few large-scale, quantitative surveys on sexual activity within the general population. However, one recent large-scale survey, the National Survey of Sexual Attitudes and Lifestyles (NSSAL) provides valuable data about sexual health within Britain.[2]

HETEROSEXUAL BEHAVIOUR
Age at first intercourse

The NSSAL asked respondents to report how old they were the first time they had sexual intercourse. For women now in their early 60s the median age at first intercourse was 21 years. The median age for today's 16–24-year-olds is 17.[2] This confirms a fall in age at first intercourse suggested elsewhere, and an increase in the proportions reporting experience before the age of 16, especially among women.[3]

Early sexual intercourse is associated with lower socio-economic status and educational level,[2,3] though this effect seems to be weakening.[2]

Sexual activity

In the NSSAL, respondents were asked how often they had had sex in the past 4 weeks (defined as oral sex, vaginal sex or anal sex). The majority reported between 4 and 10 occasions while 5% of 19-year-old women reported at least 25 occasions. Sexual activity decreased with age and length of partnership. Three-quarters of

widows and half of the single people interviewed reported no contacts in the past 4 weeks.[2]

Given the difficulties some people experience in reporting anal sex, the survey found that 14% of men and 13% of women reported ever having experienced anal intercourse, although less than 7% had experienced it in the last year. Anal sex was most frequent amongst 18–24-year-olds and those with multiple partners.[2]

Safe and unsafe sexual behaviour were measured in the National Survey of Sexual Attitudes and Lifestyles by whether respondents had reported having had two or more partners in the last year and had not used a condom with either partner.* (See Table 1).[2]

Table 1 **Unsafe sexual behaviour among adults: Britain 1990/91**

	Men %	Women %
Age group		
16–24	9.7	9.2
25–34	5.8	3.8
35–44	5.7	3.1
45–59	3.7	1.6
Marital status		
married	3.0	1.3
cohabiting	10.4	5.7
widowed/separated/divorced	15.7	8.0
single	9.6	10.6
Social class		
I, II	5.5	2.6
IIINM	5.0	5.4
IIIM	7.7	1.7
IV, V other	5.9	6.6
Homosexual partners in the last year		
0	6.0	4.0
1 or more	7.4	11.0

Base: 16 924 adults aged 16–59 who have had sexual intercourse
Source: Wellings *et al.*[2]

The highest proportions of unsafe sex were found amongst divorced, separated and widowed men; this group was more than five times more likely to report unsafe sex than those who were married. There was no obvious social class gradient with respect to the reporting of safer sex. These patterns were also evident in the HEA's Health Education Monitoring Survey.[3]

* The limitations of this definition of 'unsafe' are recognised.

Rate of partner change

The great majority of British adults have had sex with one or more partners in the last 12 months. Men report more partners than women (see Table 2).[2]

Table 2 **Number of sexual partners in the last 12 months: Britain 1990/91**

	Men %	Women %
0	13.1	13.9
1	73.0	79.4
2	8.2	4.8
3–4	4.1	1.6
5 or more	1.5	0.4

Base: 18 876 adults
Source: Wellings *et al.*[2]

This compares with 72% of women and 63% of men who had had only one sexual partner and 16% of men and 9% of women who reported two or more partners in the last year in the Health Education Monitoring Survey.[3]

Multiple partnerships tend to be associated with younger age groups.[2,3]

Men and women reporting two or more partners in the last year were more likely to be unmarried or cohabiting, to have had sex before the age of 16 and be in social classes I and II.[2]

Sexual behaviour in specific contexts

Travel

British citizens made over 31 million overseas visits in 1989; 17 million visitors were received into the UK in the same year.[4]

Surveillance data from the Communicable Diseases Surveillance Centre (CDSC) indicate that the number of HIV infections presumed to have been acquired abroad through heterosexual intercourse is increasing.[5]

Being on holiday has been thought to encourage a 'carefree attitude' to STD prevention,[6] but has not been conclusively demonstrated in studies in this area;[7–13] it is difficult to obtain representative samples of travellers to and from the UK.

Frequency of travel did not correlate with number of sexual partners in the sexual attitudes and lifestyles survey.[2]

Alcohol and drug misuse

The relationship between drug taking, sexual activity and sexual risk remains uncertain; certain drugs may increase sexual activity as well as having an effect on safer sex practice.[14,15]

Although studies have shown an association between drinking and sexual behaviour, it is often difficult to establish whether the study is demonstrating a disinhibiting effect of alcohol on subsequent sexual encounters or whether it is simply that people who drink are more likely to take other risks.[16–18] One study among young married men and women found that men who had not consumed alcohol beforehand were three times more likely to have used contraception than those who had (57% and 13% respectively, for women 68% and 24% respectively).[17]

Because HIV can be transmitted through the sharing of injecting equipment, injecting drug users are potentially a 'high-risk' group, the sexual behaviour of which could have implications for the spread of HIV.

Available evidence on injecting drug users in the UK suggests that most are in stable relationships[16,19] and that the majority are sexually active,[20,21,22] though condom usage remains low.[23,24]

In one study the majority of men and 40% of women had non-injecting partners; one-third never used condoms with casual partners.[19]

In a study of 144 under-25-year-olds who were injecting amphetamines, all respondents were sexually active and condom use was low. Respondents tended to think their HIV risk was minimal, believing that the risk of HIV infection only applied to heroin users.[19]

Although there is some evidence for a reduction in injecting risk behaviour of injecting drug users in London between 1990 and 1993, HIV transmission risk behaviour continues; needle sharing still persists, especially amongst close friends and sexual partners.[25]

Ecstasy and crack cocaine have been associated with risk of HIV infection because some users exchange sex for drugs or money.[26] Amphetamine users tended to have more casual partners and use condoms less frequently in a comparison of amphetamine and heroin users.[27]

Commercial sex workers

In a review of the sex industry, Plant *et al.*[28] concluded that heavy drinking and illicit drug use were associated with prostitution and high-risk sexual activity.

Two studies suggest that female sex workers are in the main adopting safer sexual practices. In a cross-sectional survey of 280 female sex workers in London 98% reported condom use with all clients, and 12% used condoms with non-paying partners.[29] Gossop however, found that nearly a quarter of women prostitutes interviewed were sometimes having unprotected sex with their clients.[30]

There have been suggestions that since safer sex practice is relatively high in this group, preventive strategies should be aimed at sex workers' clients who pressurise women to provide unprotected sex [31] and who may offer more money for such practices.[32]

Gossop also found that of the female sex workers interviewed with a sexual partner, 80% of their partners were also drug users and half were drug injectors. However, two-thirds of the sex workers reported never or rarely using condoms for sex with their partners.[33]

HOMOSEXUAL BEHAVIOUR

In the United Kingdom homosexual intercourse between men is the most common method of transmission of HIV – latest figures for June 1996 show that 61.1% of reports of HIV-1 infection were contracted among homosexual/bisexual men.[34] Woman-to-woman transmission of HIV is rare, and studies have shown that in cases where it has occurred other risk factors (such as injecting drug use) were nearly always known to be present.[35]

Just over 6% of men and 3.4% of women report ever having had some homosexual contact (for 3.5% of men and 1.7% of women this involved genital contact);*
1.4% of men reported having had a homosexual

* *Some definitions*
sexual contact: this is a wide term and can include just kissing and cuddling, not necessarily leading to genital contact or intercourse.
genital contact: forms of contact with the genital area not leading to intercourse (vaginal, anal or oral) but intended to achieve orgasm, for example, stimulating by hand.
sexual partner: people who have had sex together – whether just once, a few times, as regular partners or as married partners.[2]

partner in the last 5 years and 3.6% had ever had a homosexual partner: suggesting that for many people homosexuality is a passing experience.[2]

Regional differences in reporting of homosexual behaviour were striking, with 11.9% of men living in Greater London reporting that they had ever had a homosexual experience involving genital contact compared to the national average of 4.8%.[2]

Sources of information
The representativeness of the sample is a particular issue in studies of homosexual behaviour, many studies of homosexual behaviour have recruited the sample from genito-urinary medicine clinics in which homosexual men with above average sexual activity are probably over-represented. Also, the reference population in this area is not easy to define.

The National Survey of Sexual Attitudes and Lifestyles [2] does include a representative sample, but because of unwillingness to report homosexual activity, studies exclusively among gay or bisexual men or lesbians are important sources of information on homosexual behaviour.

The HEA's AIDS Research in Gay Bar Surveys, carried out every year since 1986, provide a comparable series of data on the sexual behaviour of men who attend gay bars.[36] Project SIGMA (Socio-sexual Investigations of Gay Men and AIDS) studied a cohort of 930 men from a number of sources in England and Wales from 1987 to 1993.[37]

Age at first intercourse
Estimates of average age at first intercourse for males with a man range from just under 17,[36] to just under 21.[37]

Sexual activity
The SIGMA sample provides detailed information on sexual practices among men who have sex with men.[37] Of this sample, 71% had engaged in anal intercourse in the last year, 22% were exclusively the insertive partner, 12% exclusively the receptive partner, and 43% alternated.[37] A similar pattern was found in the NSSAL.[2]

Around 40% of men who had engaged in anal intercourse in the last month had always used condoms. Men in regular relationships were less likely to use condoms; in fact most unprotected penetrative sex takes place within regular sexual relationships.[37]

While a number of studies have suggested an increase in 'unsafe' sexual practices in recent years, it remains unclear as to whether this trend is true for the whole population of homosexual men or for a minority, with the majority continuing the trend toward safer sex (see p.41).

Rate of partner change

At least one regular sexual partner plus other partners is the commonest sexual relationship configuration among gay men,[38] and the median number of sexual partners in the last year was four[37] (both SIGMA data).

In the HEA's Gay Bar Survey the median number of partners reported in the last 12 months increased from 5.4 in 1986 to 6.1 in 1996.[36]

Sexual behaviour in specific contexts

Alcohol and drug misuse

The relationship between drinking and drug use and higher-risk homosexual behaviour is debated. A three-year prospective study of 1300 homosexual men in San Francisco found 'a strong relationship between drug and alcohol use during sex and non-compliance with safer sex'.[39]

In contrast, a SIGMA study of 461 men, who reported all sexual behaviour and alcohol use in a diary format, found that alcohol use prior to or during sex was not associated with engagement in anal intercourse, casual sex or condom use.[37]

Commercial sex workers

One SIGMA study of male sex workers in South Wales found that out of 81 men in the sample, 78 had had sex with a paying partner in the month before the interview; of these the average number of partners was 31 per month. For those engaging in anal sex the average number of partners was 18. While on 84% of occasions involving receptive intercourse condoms were reportedly used, condom use was reported in only 53% of occasions with non-paying partners. The mean age of the men was 18, ranging from 15 to 23.[40]

BISEXUAL BEHAVIOUR

A recent HEA survey of behaviourally bisexual men[41] showed that 87% of those sampled had both male and female partners in the past year. Whilst the men sampled did not have as many partners as gay men,[42, 37] they had a significant number of partners and, on average, probably more female partners than the general male population.[2] While they were more likely to have regular female than regular male partners, they had roughly equal numbers of male and female partners.

Respondents were far more likely to use condoms with casual than regular partners. Overall 67.1% of respondents had engaged in unprotected vaginal intercourse and 22.6% in unprotected anal intercourse with a female, compared with less than 20% who had done so with a male.[41]

Disclosure of current sexual activities to regular female partners was not the norm, though it was to regular male partners.[41]

Most considered themselves reasonably well informed about HIV although levels of knowledge (88%) were closer to those in the general population than to the higher levels among gay men; over half displayed a correct understanding of basic concepts, including a high level of understanding about which sexual acts were most risky for HIV transmission. Those who had made changes in sexual behaviour as a consequence of HIV reported the following strategies:

- changes in sexual behaviour

- change of partner selection strategies

- increased use of condoms.[41]

ATTITUDES

Attitudes towards risk behaviour

The Health Education Monitoring Survey among adults in England in 1995[3] found that 26% of respondents (aged 16–74) thought there was no risk of ever being infected with HIV, and 59% thought the risk was low. Only 10% thought that someone like them had a 'very high' or 'quite high' risk of infection by HIV.

This compares with results from the earlier HEA Health and Lifestyles survey in 1992 among 16–54-year-olds, which asked about perceived risk of HIV from unprotected sexual intercourse. This showed that 62% of women and 65% of men felt that the average chances of getting HIV from unprotected intercourse were high.[44]

In the Health Education Monitoring Survey, a higher proportion of younger compared to older people believed they were at some risk of contracting both HIV and another STD (see Figures 1 and 2). Those with two or more partners in the last year were more likely to perceive themselves at risk. This is in keeping with results from the earlier HEA survey (but with questions restricted to HIV/AIDS) – 69% women and 70% men aged 45–54 thought their chances were less than average compared with 43% of women and 53% of men aged 16–24 years.

Nineteen per cent of women and 32% of men in the HEA's Health and Lifestyles Survey reported that they would use a condom if they had sex with a new partner,[44] though other national samples have found higher agreement. For example, in the HEA's Health Education Monitoring Survey, over half of respondents

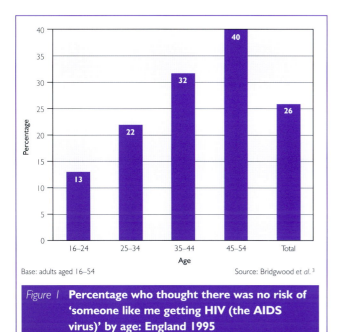

Base: adults aged 16–54   Source: Bridgwood et al. [3]

Figure 1 **Percentage who thought there was no risk of 'someone like me getting HIV (the AIDS virus)' by age: England 1995**

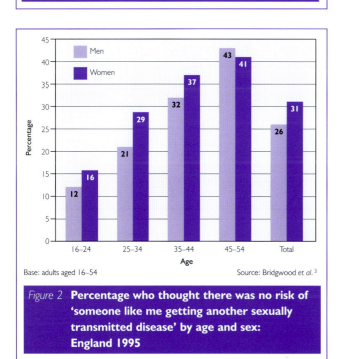

Base: adults aged 16–54   Source: Bridgwood et al. [3]

Figure 2 **Percentage who thought there was no risk of 'someone like me getting another sexually transmitted disease' by age and sex: England 1995**

(64% of women and 54% of men) said that 'if in the near future, they did have sex with a new partner, 'they would always use a condom'.[3]

The Health Education Monitoring Survey also asked questions about attitudes towards safer sex. Despite the results showing low perceived risk, almost all (96%) respondents believed that 'using condoms would show that someone was a responsible person'; 95% believed that 'condoms would protect against unwanted pregnancy'; and 95% 'strongly agreed' or 'agreed' that 'using condoms would protect against HIV'.[3]

However, less than a third of respondents (30% of men and 24% of women) had changed their behaviour because of concern about AIDS. The most common changes were:

● using condoms (15% of men, 11% of women)

● sticking to one partner (12% of men, 11% of women)

● finding out more about someone before having sex (10% of men, 9% of women).[3]

Seventy per cent of men in the Gay Bar Survey who said they practice safer sex all the time say direct experience of seeing the effect of AIDS on members of the gay community was a key factor in changing behaviour; AIDS educational campaigns and editorial coverage had also had an effect.[36]

Attitudes towards homosexuality

Because gay and bisexual men in this country have been the most affected by HIV and AIDS, and AIDS has been viewed as a 'homosexual disease', examination of the public's attitudes towards homosexuality is relevant. Latest available statistics show that in 1991:

● 67% of adults aged 16+ in the UK agree with the statement 'On the whole, I am tolerant of homosexuality'

● 83% agree that 'Homosexual men should be judged on their personal merits just like everyone else – what they do in private is their own business'

● 58% would not be embarrassed if they learnt that one of their relatives was homosexual.

However, 65% of adults believe that scenes showing homosexual relationships should be banned from television and films. There has been little change in these attitudes since tracking began in 1988.[43]

YOUNG ADULTS
Age at first intercourse
Fifty-two per cent of all 16–19-year-olds have had sexual intercourse,[45] a finding similar to that in the HEA's Health Education Monitoring Survey in which 57% reported having had a sexual partner.[3]

Table 3 **Young adults (16–19) who have had sexual intercourse: England 1990**

Age	Men %	Women %
16	31	31
17	45	42
18	60	61
19	70	70
all (16–19)	52	52

Base: 4436 16–19-year-olds
Source: HEA[45]

Young Asians are less likely to report having had sexual intercourse (24%) than their white (53%) and Afro-Caribbean peers (51%). Similarly, young people from socioeconomic group AB households are slightly less likely to have had full sexual intercourse (47%) than those from households in social groups C, D and E (see Appendix 1 for definition of social classes).[45]

Findings from a large survey of 3777 16–24-year-olds in the south-west of England, show 41% of all ages reporting that they had full sexual intercourse before the age of 16.[46]

Sexual activity
Sixty-five per cent of the teenagers interviewed in the HEA's Young Adults Survey of 4436 16–19-year-olds reported that they were sexually active: of these 79% reported having had sexual intercourse. Sixty-four per cent had engaged in mutual masturbation, and 49% in oral sex. Thirty-five per cent said they were not sexually active.[45]

Three per cent of teenagers surveyed in the south-west of England considered that that they had had a homosexual experience. Nearly all respondents (95.5%) considered themselves heterosexual, 1.5% considered themselves bisexual, 0.9% considered themselves homosexual and 2.1% were not sure.[46]

Rate of partner change
One view of teenage sexual relationships is that serial monogamy* is more descriptive of the sexual lifestyles of most teenagers than one of simultaneous multiple partners.[47] In two significant surveys of young adults most (75–82%) reported that their last sexual partner was a regular or steady partner.[45, 46] However, in the south-west about a quarter of those reporting that they were in a steady relationship had had multiple partners in the last year, indicating that young people's steady relationships are not necessarily monogamous,[46] and the NSSAL found that 20.7% of 16–24 year-olds reported having had 2 or more partners in the last year.[2]

Table 4 **Number of partners with whom full sexual intercourse had taken place in the last 12 months (16–19-year-olds): England 1990**

	Men %	Women %
1	70	47
2	18	20
3	5	10
4	3	7
5–10	1	7
more than 10	<0.5	3
don't know	3	6

Base: all those who have had sexual intercourse (2158)
Source: HEA[45]

Attitudes and perceptions
Most (60–70%) young adults consider sex outside a regular relationship to be wrong.[2]

Most young people are reasonably well informed about safer sex although most would welcome more and better information.[48] When asked if they agreed with the statement 'I would be too embarrassed to suggest using a condom with a new partner', 59% of respondents in the HEA's Young Adults survey disagreed and 15% agreed.[45] Comparable results were found among 16–24-year-olds in the Health Education Monitoring Survey.[3]

This survey also found the following among 16–24-year-olds:

● 95% agreed or strongly agreed that 'using condoms would show that someone was a responsible person.'

● 62% 'would always use a condom' if in the near future they did have sex with a new partner.

* one relationship beginning after another one has finished.

When 879 18-year-olds in Glasgow were asked to give a definition of safer sex, 84% mentioned using condoms, 68% mentioned some aspect of choice of partner and 2% mentioned abstaining from specific activities. Those of a higher economic status were more likely to have a better knowledge of safer sex (defined as mentioning condom use plus one or more risk reduction strategies).[49]

Sixty-four per cent of male and 50% of female teenagers in a survey of 3777 16–24 year-olds in the south-west of England said they were less likely to use condoms after drinking.[46]

Health consequences of early sexual activity

Early teenage sexual activity may bear certain health consequences in later life:

- exposure to gonorrhoea and other sexually transmitted diseases which are most common among people in their late teens and early twenties.[50] Of people with heterosexually acquired AIDS in the UK, 31.9% are in their twenties, most of whom will (assuming a 10-year incubation period) have contracted HIV in their teens.[5]

- possible risks of developing cervical cancer in later life associated with early first intercourse.[51]

Conceptions

INTRODUCTION

There were 801 600 recorded conceptions in England and Wales in 1994.[1]

Conception statistics are derived by combining registration records of both live and still births with records of legal terminations under the Abortion Act 1967. Miscarriages or illegal abortions are not recorded centrally and thus are not included in these statistics.

Health of the Nation targets

The Government's *Health of the Nation* White Paper suggests that 'it is reasonable to make the general assumption that pregnancies in those under 16 years of age are not wanted'.[2]

The general *Health of the Nation* objectives are to reduce the number of unwanted pregnancies and ensure effective family planning services for people who want them.

Specific objectives are to reduce the rate of conceptions among under-16s by at least 50% by the year 2000 (to no more than 4.8 per 1000 in under 16-year-old women).

Broadening access to family planning services, developing alliances between relevant local bodies and ensuring the availability of comprehensive and effective sex education for young people were also discussed.

Surveys suggest that between one-third and one-half of conceptions are unintended.[3-5] However, the Royal College of Obstetricians and Gynaecologists have made clear that '*an unintended or unplanned pregnancy could become wanted and the term "unwanted" does not convey the ambivalence felt by women who become pregnant unintentionally. Unwanted pregnancies are usually but not always unplanned. The main factors that make a pregnancy unwanted are the woman's personal feelings and the social and economic circumstances of her life: critically, her relationship with her partner*'.[6]

TEENAGE CONCEPTIONS

Conceptions among teenagers are of particular concern. Between 50% and 90% of teenage pregnancies are unintended,[5,7,8] and among those under 16 years of age, 52.8% of conceptions led to abortion in 1994.[1] Teenage pregnancy has policy implications for the provision of contraceptive services and sex education.

In addition, there are adverse health consequences of early teenage sexual activity and pregnancy. These are:

● Children of teenage mothers may be at higher risk of a variety of conditions such as prematurity, low birthweight, congenital malformations,[9, 10] and risk of sudden infant death syndrome.[11] However, much of this risk may be due to the social and financial circumstances of young mothers and inadequate antenatal care,[12] rather than teenage childbearing per se.[13]

● risks associated with late termination of pregnancy. Pregnant teenagers are more likely to have a late abortion (over 20 weeks gestation) than women aged 20 or above.[14] This may reflect delays in the discovery of pregnancy and/or knowledge/access to the appropriate services.[15]

Figure 3 shows trends in conception rates among women under 20 between 1984 and 1994.

Table 5   **Teenage pregnancy: England and Wales 1994**

Number: 85 000 teenage conceptions
Rates:
Under 20:   58.6 per 1000 females aged 15–19.
Under 16:   8.3 per 1000 females aged 13–15.
Trends:
Under 20:   Conception rates increased from 59 per 1000 in 1980, peaking at 69 per 1000 in 1990, but have declined significantly since, down to 58.6 per 1000 women in 1994.
Under 16:   Conception rates increased from 7.2 per 1000 in 1980, peaking at 10.1 in 1990 but thereafter declined to 8.1 per 1000 women in 1993. In 1994, there was a slight increase to 8.3 per 1000 women.
Conceptions leading to maternities:
Under 20:   64.7% led to maternities.
Under 16:   47.2% led to maternities.

Source: ONS[1]

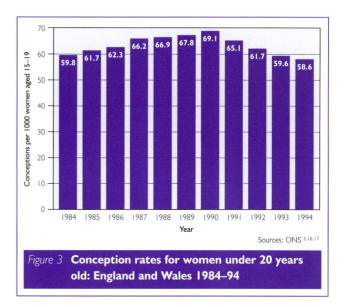

Sources: ONS [3,16,17]

Figure 3   **Conception rates for women under 20 years old: England and Wales 1984–94**

International comparisons

Within Europe, Eastern European countries have the highest teenage birth rates, though Britain has the highest rates among Western European countries. Birth rates are used as a proxy measure for conception rates.

Table 6   **Birth rates per 1000 women aged under 20 years: Europe**

Bulgaria	(1993)	67.3
Russia	(1990)	55.6
Turkey	(1994)	53.0
Romania	(1994)	45.0
Czech Republic	(1993)	42.9p
Hungary	(1994)	33.6
England and Wales*	(1995)	28.9
Scotland*	(1995)	28.3
Poland	(1994)	25.5
Northern Ireland*	(1995)	27.2
Austria	(1994)	18.9
Portugal	(1994)	21.2
Greece	(1994)	14.2
Norway	(1994)	14.4
Germany	(1993)	11.8
Sweden	(1994)	9.6
Spain	(1992)	10.3
Denmark	(1993)	8.8
France	(1992)	8.7
Italy	(1992)	7.6
Netherlands	(1993)	5.4
Switzerland	(1994)	4.0

Source: Council of Europe [18]

* ONS Fertility Statistics Unit, 1996.   p provisional

International differences in teenage birth rates (used as a proxy for conception rates) cannot be accounted for by differences in sexual activity. A multivariate analysis found that the following correlated with low adolescent birth rates:

● High GNP per capita

● favourable income distribution

● high proportion of the population foreign born

● high percentage of the population living in large cities

● high minimum age at marriage without parental consent

● openness about sex

● high percentage of women taught about contraception in schools

● Government policy to provide contraceptives to the young.[19]

The UK teenage birth rate is five times the rate in the Netherlands. The Netherlands' success has been attributed to a network of specialist youth clinics with a reputation for providing non-moralistic, confidential client-centred services.[20]

Aspects of family planning provision which are considered important determinants of quality in the UK, family planning trained practice nurses for example, are not strong features of Dutch family planning services; this may suggest that a sexual culture which encourages teenagers to ask for and use contraception is as important as issues of access and quality of services.[20]

Regional variations
Teenage conception rates vary between and within regions in the UK. The lowest conception rates among teenagers are found in the south, with some of the highest rates in the north (see Figure 4).[1]

Districts with high underprivileged area scores were more likely to have high rates of conception among teenagers in an analysis of districts in the former North East Thames region.[23] Teenage conception rates are also higher in inner cities and other urban areas.[14]

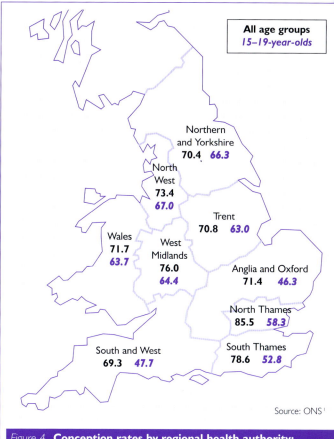

All age groups
15–19-year-olds

Northern and Yorkshire
70.4 66.3

North West
73.4 67.0

Trent
70.8 63.0

Wales
71.7 63.7

West Midlands
76.0 64.4

Anglia and Oxford
71.4 46.3

North Thames
85.5 58.3

South and West
69.3 47.7

South Thames
78.6 52.8

Source: ONS[1]

Figure 4 **Conception rates by regional health authority: England and Wales 1994**

Socioeconomic group
Data from some national surveys show that highest levels of teenage births occur to the most socio-economically disadvantaged women.[14]

Teenage birth rates among manual social classes were 3 times the rate found among non-manual classes for two cohorts of women born in 1957–61 and 1964–68 and for whom births were linked to census information in a longitudinal study conducted by the Office of Population Censuses and Surveys. A similar pattern was shown when the women were classified according to housing tenure and car ownership, with the highest birth rate occurring to women in local authority accommodation with no access to a car.[14]

Teenage mothers are more likely than older mothers to have left school early, to be born among larger families and to be born to a teenage mother themselves.[7,21,22]

However, an important factor influencing the prevalence of teenage motherhood is whether the pregnancy is continued or terminated. Although nationally and in more affluent areas abortion is the main outcome of pregnancies in girls under 16, in more urban areas the main outcome is maternity. Studies show that the proportion of teenage pregnancies ending in abortion is higher in more affluent areas whereas women who are more socioeconomically disadvantaged tend to continue with their pregnancy.[7, 14, 23]

Financial cost

Information on the costs to the NHS of unwanted pregnancies in the UK is difficult to obtain and not comprehensive. As more work is undertaken on the effectiveness and cost-effectiveness of health promotion, more information should become available.

One report looking at the cost-effectiveness of family planning services, by the Contraceptive Alliance, claims that 3 million unplanned pregnancies in Britain are avoided per year by the use of family planning services, representing a saving of over £2.5 billion per year to the NHS (this includes abortion costs).[24] Moreover, if the costs of claiming income maintenance and the cost of maintaining a child to age 16 are taken into account it is claimed that £22.5 billion was saved in 1991.

The figure of 3 million unplanned pregnancies in Britain per year may be an overestimate. It is calculated in the report by estimating the number of current users of all ages of each form of contraception and information on the effectiveness of each form of contraception. This is relative to the use of no method of contraception. There are approximately 10 million women aged 15–44 in England and there were 648 000 live births in 1995.[25] Moreover, an 'unplanned' pregnancy is not necessarily an unwanted pregnancy. Abortions can be taken as a proxy measure of unwanted pregnancy; there were 163 621 abortions in England and Wales in 1995.[26]

Contraception

INTRODUCTION

The period between the early 1960s and the mid-1970s saw a marked decline in mechanical methods of contraception and a dramatic increase in the use of hormonal methods. Since the mid-1970s the trend has been away from the pill towards sterilisation and in the 1980s towards the condom.[1–5]

While in the 1960s and 1970s availability of contraception was an important determinant of use, in the 1980s and 1990s considerations of efficacy, safety and acceptability are now the main determinants of contraceptive use.

USE OF CONTRACEPTION

In the 1991 and 1993 OPCS General Household Surveys (GHS),[5] over 5000 women were asked which, if any, of the list of contraceptive methods they and their partner had used in the last year, and which they 'usually use at present' (see Figure 5). In 1993, questions were asked on emergency contraception.

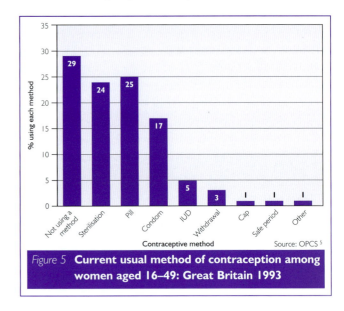

Figure 5 **Current usual method of contraception among women aged 16–49: Great Britain 1993**

In 1993, 29% of women and their partners were not using any method of contraception. The most common cited reasons included abstinence or no sexual partner (15%), pregnancy (3%) or trying to get pregnant (5%), and sterility after an operation. Figures do not add up to 100% as women may use more than one method of contraception or give more than one reason for not using contraception.[5]

In a smaller but more recent survey of 1000 women aged 16–44, 1 in 3 women reported using the pill and 1 in 5, the condom.[6]

Trends

Figure 6 reflects trends in contraceptive use observed between 1983 and 1993.[4]

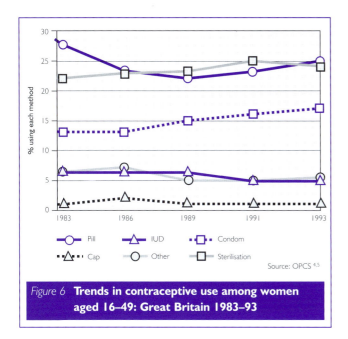

Figure 6 **Trends in contraceptive use among women aged 16–49: Great Britain 1983–93**

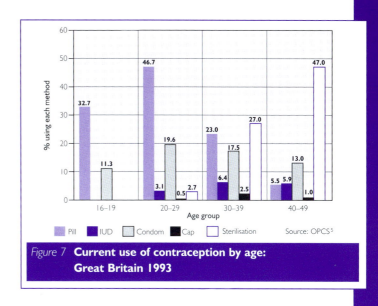

Figure 7 **Current use of contraception by age: Great Britain 1993**

However, figures for 1983 are not strictly comparable with figures for later years; since 1983 the age band included in the survey has widened from all women aged 18–44 to all women aged 16–49. Over this decade, there was little change in the proportion of women using no method of contraception in each survey year.

Use of the pill has declined from 28% of 18–44-year-old women using this method in 1983 to 25% in 1993.

Between 1986 and 1993, the proportion of women whose partners used the condom rose from 13% to 17%. This was predominantly among women under 30, with the largest increase among partners of women aged 18–19 years (from 6% to 22%). Among younger women aged 16–17 years, an increase in condom use was reported much later, between 1991 and 1993, when usage rose significantly from 10 to 17%.

Age group

Figure 7 shows the proportions of each age group who report usually using any of the methods of contraception listed. In the National Survey of Sexual Attitudes and Lifestyles,[7] more than 9 out of 10 sexually active 16–24-year-old men and women reported the use of at least one method of contraception in the past year compared to two-thirds of men and just over half of women aged 45–59 years, many of whom will no longer be of child-bearing age.

Socioeconomic group

Contraceptive use varies by social class. The National Survey of Sexual Attitudes and Lifestyles found the association with social class to be more marked for whether a method is used than for the type of method chosen.

Ethnic group

Although sexual health data relating to different ethnic groups are scarce, patterns of contraceptive use and attitudes to contraception have been documented, mostly among Asian communities.[9–12]

Health Education Authority research data on 1017 Indians, 927 Pakistanis and 665 Bangladeshis found that all 3 groups were more likely than the general population to have used a condom or an IUD at last sexual intercourse. Asians were less likely than the general population to have used no contraception at last intercourse.[12]

A survey of 501 randomly selected Asian women in Leicester found that the most popular contraceptive methods were the IUD (33%), the condom (31%) and the pill (26%), as compared to GHS figures for the national population of 5%, 17% and 25% respectively.[9,5] Although variations in contraceptive use between religious groups was apparent, religion did not appear to be a barrier to accepting or using contraception.[9]

However, in the National Survey of Sexual Attitudes and Lifestyles,[7] religion showed a weak association with contraceptive use. Those of non-Christian religion were most likely to have used no method at all compared with those of other religious denominations; they were nearly twice as likely to use no method as those with no religious denomination, among whom reports of no method use were the lowest.

Table 7 **Main method of contraception by social class*: England and Wales 1991**

Current method of contraception	Social class						Total %
	A %	B %	C1 %	C2 %	D %	E %	
Pill	30.8	31.7	37.0	38.7	42.6	42.3	38.3
IUD	3.8	4.9	5.4	7.9	9.2	8.1	7.1
Condom	34.6	27.3	29.0	19.6	21.6	21.1	23.8
Diaphragm	7.7	4.4	1.9	1.3	0.4	0.8	1.7
Sterilisation (total)	23.1	27.3	25.0	28.7	24.2	22.8	26.1
Female sterilisation	(7.7)	(10.9)	(10.4)	(13.5)	(13.3)	(18.3)	(12.6)
Male sterilisation	(15.4)	(16.4)	(14.6)	(15.2)	(10.9)	(4.5)	(13.5)
Natural methods	0.0	3.3	0.9	2.7	1.4	0.8	1.9
Injection	0.0	0.5	–	0.4	0.4	2.4	0.4
Other	–	0.5	0.7	0.8	–	1.6	0.6

Base: 1570   * See Appendix 1 for definitions   Source: Blacksell *et al.*[8]

USE, KNOWLEDGE AND ATTITUDES TOWARDS SPECIFIC METHODS
All adults
In a survey of over 2000 adults aged 18–44, 89% thought that contraception should be the joint responsibility of both men and women.[8]

Oral contraceptives
Use of oral contraceptives ('the pill') is most common among single, cohabiting women and women with no children. Of those using a contraceptive method, 28% of married or cohabiting women as opposed to 67% of single women use the pill as their main method of contraception.[5]

The decrease in popularity of the pill may have been in response to studies linking pill use to increased risk of cardiovascular disease in 1977,[13,14] and breast and cervical cancer in 1983.[15,16]

Modern hormone dosages differ considerably from the pill dosages observed in these studies; more favourable reporting of outcomes of modern pill usage could reverse this trend.[17]

Amongst women who become pregnant on the pill, only a small minority of cases are considered to be due to method failure. Most unintended pregnancies are due to missed pills or medical complications such as vomiting or diarrhoea.[18]

Two studies, one with a sample size of 733 women undergoing termination of pregnancy and the other of 40 women randomly selected from attendances at family planning clinics, have identified significant gaps in pill users' knowledge of what to do if a pill is missed or a medical complication occurs.[19,20] When asked 'in which situation might the pill not work?' approximately half of the pill users in two family planning clinics did not know of any of the factors which lessen the pill's effectiveness.[20]

In surveys of contraceptive use, a change from another form of contraception to the pill has been associated with the transition from a casual to a more permanent relationship.[8,21]

In October 1995, the Committee on Safety of Medicines announced that 'combined oral contraceptives containing destrogel and gestodene . . . are associated with around a two-fold increase in the risk of thrombo-embolism'.[22] Though the excess risk of thromboembolism is still comparatively small, it was estimated that 12% of women on the affected pills were sufficiently concerned that they stopped using the pill.[23] Though the impact of the pill scare in terms of unplanned pregnancies and consequent abortions has yet to be assessed, estimates suggest that the overall increase in abortions may be as high as 3000.[24]

The intrauterine device (IUD)
The intrauterine device became more popular in the late 1970s following disaffection with the pill. Later adverse

reports linking the IUD with pelvic inflammatory disease and the withdrawal of one make of IUD (the Dalkon Shield™) reversed this trend. The slightly higher risk of infertility associated with the IUD means that it is not popular (and generally not recommended) among younger women,[25] although IUDs are popular amongst Asians.

The cap and diaphragm
Female barrier methods are very much a minority method and are becoming increasingly so. Diaphragm use is 7 times as common among professionals as among people in manual occupations.[8]

The condom
Condom use has become more frequent in recent years (Figure 8), and while condoms have become more socially acceptable[8] only very small proportions of people taking up the condom as their main method of contraception do so for protection from HIV.[26,8]

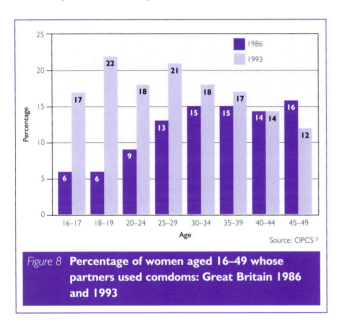

Figure 8 **Percentage of women aged 16–49 whose partners used comdoms: Great Britain 1986 and 1993**

In the 1993, GHS 17% of women cited the (male) condom as their usual method of contraception, and 9% reported having changed from some other method to the condom.[5] Other surveys suggest that anxieties about the risks and side effects of the pill are the most common reason for changing to condom use.[27,8]

Condom users are more likely to be single or married women (as opposed to divorced, widowed or cohabiting women) and under 30 years of age. This reflects the increase in condom use since 1991, predominantly among 16–17-year-olds, described earlier. This marks a change since 1991 when condom use was most popular among those aged 35–44 years.

However, the popularity of condoms declines beyond 30 years of age.[5]

Similar trends with age were found among men and women in the National Survey of Sexual Attitudes and Lifestyles[7] and in the Health Education Monitoring Survey (HEMS), a national survey of adults aged 16–74 years.[28]

In a national population-based survey of over 2000 adults, condom use was most frequent amongst 26–30-year-olds, married or cohabiting women (63% of current users) and professional and white-collar social groups.[8] (Variations in reported condom use may reflect differences in how the question was put.)

Condom users are also more likely to be socio-economically classified under non-manual status, and to have the highest qualifications. (Male use of condoms is not reported in the GHS because only women are asked about contraceptive use.)[5]

Sterilisation
Sterilisation is the preferred method of contraception among women who have completed their families. Female sterilisation is inversely related to social class and educational level.[5,8]

New methods
New and future hormonal contraceptive methods include implants, hormone-releasing vaginal rings, contraceptive skin patches, nasal sprays, vaccines and male hormonal methods.[26]

The female condom has aroused considerable interest; early testing suggests that it is not popular amongst most couples although it is acceptable amongst a small minority.[29] Further studies have found that after 3 months of use the majority of women felt generally positive about the method and 41% intended to use it in the future, although this was a relatively motivated population and may not be representative of the population of women as a whole.[30]

A study among 79 women who used the female condom for the first time showed it to be an acceptable form of contraception to 69% of women and 45% of men, with 33% of women and 10% of men finding sexual pleasure with the female condom to be the same or better than no barrier method at all.[31]

The female condom is made of polyurethane which is stronger than latex rubber.

Young adults

In the Health Education Monitoring Survey,[28] a national survey of 16–74-year-olds carried out by the HEA, 86% of 16–19-year-old men and 91% of 16–19-year-old women used at least one method of contraception at first intercourse, mainly the condom and the pill (79% and 13% of respondents respectively). Six per cent subsequently used emergency contraceptives on that occasion.

In the same survey, when asked about the method used on the last occasion of intercourse, 50% of 16–24-year-olds reported using the pill and 43% the condom.

Another survey carried out in the south-west of England found 28% of young adults between the ages of 16 and 24 reported not having used any method of contraception at last intercourse. Thirty-six per cent of the sample reported having used hormonal methods, and 5%, hormonal methods and the condom.[21]

In an earlier study carried out by the HEA among 16–19-year-olds, 8% of young women and 7% of young men reported that they had not used any form of contraception the last time they had intercourse.[32]

Table 8 **Type of contraception used by either partner at last intercourse amongst teenagers and young adults aged 16–24: England 1995**

	Women %	Men %
Condom	32	55
Pill	58	41
Other (including sterilisation)	3	2
Emergency contraception	3	2
Female condom	1	–
None	12	6
Don't know/can't remember	1	3

Base: All who reported a sexual partner in the last year (2472)
Figures do not add up to 100% as more than one method may have been used.
Source: HEA[28]

The younger teenagers are at first intercourse, the less likely they are to use contraception[7,33] although this trend is not supported by the study in the south-west mentioned above.[21]

Younger teenagers and teenagers from middle-class backgrounds are more likely to use condoms than older teenagers or those from less advantaged socioeconomic backgrounds. The most important considerations cited by teenagers in their choice of contraception (in order of frequency) are: prevention of pregnancy, prevention of risk from AIDS, prevention of risk of infection from other diseases and ease of use.[32]

In the survey in the south-west, unprotected intercourse was most likely to take place outside of the steady relationship. Condom use was strongly endorsed by a third of the respondents; only 8% said that they 'would not use a condom because the risk of HIV infection was so low'.[21]

Sixty-four per cent of male and 50% of female teenagers in a survey of 3777 16–24-year-olds in the south-west of England said they were less likely to use condoms after drinking.[21]

The latest GHS showed that between 1986 and 1993, condoms became more popular among partners of young women in the 18–19 year age group: from 6 to 22% in 1986 and 1993 respectively. Among 16–17-year-olds, there was a dramatic increase in reported condom use from 10 to 17% between 1991 and 1993.[5]

Confidentiality and the law

In 1985 the House of Lords ruling in the Gillick case established the current legal position in England and Wales: people under 16 who are fully able to understand what is proposed and its implications are competent to consent to medical treatment regardless of age. So long as this condition is fulfilled doctors are obliged to encourage teenagers who want contraception to seek parental consent but are not obliged to inform the parents themselves of their child's intentions.[34] Doctors are under the same duty of confidentiality as they are for patients over the age of 16.

EFFECTIVENESS OF CONTRACEPTIVE METHODS

As yet no contraceptive method is completely protective simultaneously against sexually transmitted diseases (STDs) and pregnancy. Many studies have shown a protective effect of barrier methods and spermicide against STDs but most studies have been conducted amongst high risk-groups or *in vitro* and are not representative therefore of the general population.

Protection against pregnancy

Table 9 summarises failure rates by type of contraceptive for preventing pregnancy. The figures indicate that while sterilisation is the most effective intervention in

Table 9 **Failure rates by type of contraceptive for preventing pregnancy**

Method of contraception	Failure rate per 100 women per year	Comments
Combined pill	<1 (careful use) 3 or more (less careful)	Forgetfulness or irregular pill taking is the major cause of failure. Up to 53% of users do not take pill regularly.[36]
Progestogen-only pill	<1 (careful use) 4 or more (less careful)	Failure is mainly due to non-compliance. Protection may also be lost by the use of other drugs.[37]
Injectable contraceptive	<1	
IUD	<1–2	Pregnancy rate depends on type of device, age of woman, parity and duration of use. Use of spermicide increases efficacy.[38]
Implant	<1 (first year) 2 (over the 5 years of use)	
Male condom (latex)	2 (careful use) 2–15 (less careful)	Effectiveness is increased with use of spermicide. Should be used with water-based lubricants.
Female condom	5 (careful) 21 (less careful)	Initial research suggests the female condom ought to be as effective as the male.[39,40]
Diaphragm or cap with spermicide	4–8 (careful use) 10–18 (less careful)	
Natural methods (symptothermal method)	2 (careful) 2–20 (less careful)	Methods may fail due to being complicated, too difficult to apply, and having too many rules to remember.[38]
Intrauterine system	<1	
Female sterilisation	1–3 per 1000	Depends on method used.
Male sterilisation	1 per 1000	Additional contraception is needed until 2 consequent sperm counts have been obtained showing no sperm present.

Source: UK Family Planning Association [35]

preventing pregnancy, the most effective 'non-permanent' methods are the intrauterine system, injectable hormones and hormonal implants, followed by the pill. Of every 100 women using the pill according to instructions, less than 1% will become pregnant in a year.[35]

Reliability of condoms is variable – a study by the Consumers' Association found that 9 brands out of 34 failed a series of rigorous tests to assess strength and to check for presence of holes.[41]

Contraceptives are likely to be less effective if not used according to instructions.

Protection against HIV infection and sexually transmitted diseases
Condoms
Laboratory studies show that intact latex condoms provide a continuous mechanical barrier to hepatitis B virus, *Chlamydia trachomatis* and *Neisseria gonorrhoea* as well as HIV.[42] Natural membrane condoms are less effective – hepatitis B surface antigens are able to pass through natural membrane condoms but not through latex condoms.[43]

Current evidence from human studies also indicates that condom use may reduce the rate of sexually transmitted HIV. An aggregated estimate of condom effectiveness suggests a 69% reduction in risk, but true 'in-use' effectiveness may be as low as 46% or as high as 82%. Thus it is correct to say that condoms reduce the risk of HIV transmission rather than prevent it.[44]

A growing body of evidence also shows that condom use reduces the risk for gonorrhoea, herpes simplex virus infection, genital ulcers and pelvic inflammatory disease, although different studies show varying levels of protection.[42] However, a Finnish study found that condoms have no protective effect for women against human papilloma virus (HPV) infections.[45]

Initial studies have shown the female condom to be stronger than the male condom; unlike latex, polyurethane is resistant to oils,[46] while having comparable properties against gases, viruses and *trichomona vaginalis*.[47] Laboratory *in vitro* tests with female condoms show no leakage of HIV or cytomegalovirus. However, it seems that vaginal bacterial flora may change with use of the female condom which in turn may cause urinary tract infection.[48]

Spermicides

Studies have shown that contraceptive spermicides kill or inactivate most STD pathogens including HIV *in vitro*.

In clinical studies spermicides have also been shown to be effective against some STDs. A study in Alabama found that over 6 months, regular use of nonoxynol-9 gel by women reduced the incidence of cervical gonococcal infections by 24% and that of cervical chlamydial infections by 22%.[49] Other studies have shown protection against pelvic inflammatory disease,[50] but HPV does not appear to be affected by nonoxynol-9.[51] Studies have found that spermicides can cause irritation in some individuals with frequent use, with adverse implications for the transmission of STDs.[52]

The diaphragm and contraceptive sponge

Four case-control studies found that women who used diaphragms (with spermicide) were at least 50% less likely than those who used no method to have cervical gonorrhoea,[53] trichomoniasis,[54] tubal infertility or to be hospitalised for pelvic inflammatory disease.[50] However, diaphragms do not appear to protect against cervical human papilloma virus or herpes simplex in women.[55] Contraceptive sponges, no longer available in the UK, have been found to decrease the risk of contracting cervical gonorrhoea and cervical chlamydia but to increase the risk of vaginal yeast infection (candidiasis).[56]

Oral contraceptives

The effect of oral contraceptives on transmission, acquisition or disease progression of HIV is unclear.

The influence of oral contraceptives on other STDs is also unclear although there may be a protective effect against pelvic inflammatory disease.[42]

The intrauterine device

It was thought in the past that use of intrauterine devices led to an increased risk of pelvic inflammatory disease. This risk is now thought to have been exaggerated, but the precise effect of IUD use on the risk of infection is not known.[42] An Expert Advisory Group on Chlamydia Trachomatis established by the Department of Health in 1996 will consider recommendations for the Chief Medical Officer on the issue of screening and treatment of IUD clients for chlamydia.

Sterilisation

Sterilisation provides no protection against acquisition of bacterial or viral STDs in the lower genital tract; however tubal sterilisation in women appears to reduce the risk of pelvic inflammatory disease.[42]

In summary, condoms alone, spermicide alone, and a combination of condoms and spermicide, all provide good protection against most STDs. The condom, as a single method, provides the best overall protection against herpes, chlamydia, hepatitis B, gonorrhoea and HIV, although the evidence of effectiveness for women is more equivocal than for men.[42]

EMERGENCY CONTRACEPTION

The need for access to information and services about emergency contraception is demonstrated in abortion statistics (see next chapter) and data on unplanned pregnancies.

A survey of women in 1989, who had recently had a child, found that 31% had become pregnant unintentionally.[57]

One study showed 93% of women requesting abortion would have preferred emergency contraception to an unplanned pregnancy.[58] Seventy per cent of women requesting abortion in a 1990 study would have used emergency contraception but did not know how to get it and a further 30% were unaware of emergency contraception as an option.[59]

Emergency contraception is available as:

● the combined oestrogen and progestogen pill, which has been shown to be safe and effective if begun within 72 hours of unprotected intercourse; 2 tablets are taken within 72 hours followed by 2 tablets 12 hours later.

- the IUD. This has been shown to be safe and effective if used within 5 days of unprotected intercourse or within 5 days of calculated ovulation.

A number of studies have shown that there is a growing awareness of the existence of emergency contraception[59] but that knowledge of the time period during which the methods can be used and the range of places from which they can be obtained is low. Awareness of using an IUD for emergency contraception is poor. Only around 3% of approximately 798 women aged 16–49 years surveyed by the HEA in 1996 knew it can be fitted up to 120 hours after unprotected intercourse.

The same survey found that 97% of respondents were aware of the so-called 'morning after pill' but 75% did not know the time period after unprotected sex in which it could be used. Only 24% of respondents identified the correct time limit;[60] 14% in a smaller study.[61] In this study, nearly half of women surveyed thought that emergency contraception had to be taken within 24 hours of unprotected intercourse.

Awareness of the correct time period for using emergency contraception appears to be higher among younger women.[62] Since the majority of women who seek abortions are over 25 years of age, the education of older women is particularly important.

Use and access
The 1993 General Household Survey showed that around 5% of women aged 16–49 had used emergency contraception over the past two years, and 1% of women had used it on more than one occasion. Usage was highest among 18–24-year-olds. The majority had used the pill (96%), while 4% had had an IUD fitted.[5]

The Health Education Authority Monitoring Survey (HEMS) among 4672 adults aged 16–74 in England showed that among 278 respondents who had first sexual intercourse in the five years prior to interview, 4% reported having subsequently used emergency contraception on this first occasion.[28]

A more recent survey by the HEA in 1996 showed that 14% of women had used emergency contraception in their lives. Users tended to be young (23% among

16–24-year-olds) and more likely to be sexually active before 16 years of age, with multiple partners in the last year.[60]

In a study among 1206 14–16-year-olds in Scotland, one-third of sexually active girls aged under 16 in Lothian had used emergency contraceptives. Though 93% were aware of emergency contraception, knowledge of correct time limits was poor.[63]

Community pharmacists dispensed more than 300 000 GP prescriptions for emergency contraceptive pills in 1991.[64]

Of 126 GPs who responded to a survey conducted in 1994 by the Family Planning Association, 124 (98%) prescribed emergency contraception; 91% were willing to prescribe contraceptive pills as an emergency method; 44% postcoital IUDs. Fewer hospital accident and emergency departments had prescribed emergency contraception.[65]

Another survey showed that most genitourinary clinics (71.5%) provided emergency contraceptive pills, and 17% provided IUDs.[66]

Public perceptions of availability of emergency contraception may present a barrier to its use. The greatest concern of women who might consider using it in future was access to a GP in time, reflected in reported experience by 10% of women who had tried to use emergency contraception. Women were also concerned about issues of confidentiality with their GP.[67]

FAMILY PLANNING
General practitioners are the most common source of family planning services; more patients than before are relying on their GP than are attending family planning clinics.[8]

In a survey of 1570 16–43-year-olds in 1991, 73% mentioned GPs as the first place they would think of to go for contraceptive advice. This figure was up 7.8% from a similar survey in 1985. Family planning clinics were cited by 32% of respondents. Although family planning clinics were cited as the first place thought of for supplies, most people obtained contraceptive advice and supplies from their GP.[8]

In a survey of 167 pregnant teenagers, 92% knew where to obtain contraceptives and contraceptive advice[68] and 60% had seen their GP about contraceptive advice, compared to 30% who had attended a family planning clinic. Overall there was a high satisfaction with the service. Issues of confidentiality and approachability of the staff were cited as criticisms of GP services, while better advertising, accessibility and improved privacy were cited as advantages of family planning clinics.

Table 10 **Family planning services in England – numbers of patients seen by different providers**

1988/89	1993/94	1994/95
Community and hospital clinics		
1 204 000	1 110 000	1 152 000
(Each person counted at first visit to clinic in a district during the year)		
Family health services		
2 658 900	2 948 900	–
(Number of patients at the end of the year in respect of whom a fee is payable to a GP for providing contraceptive services)		

Source: DoH[69]

Family planning clinic users tend to be young women delaying childbearing or women who wish to stop childbearing. Women attending GP surgeries for family planning are more likely to be currently spacing their pregnancies.[70]

GPs prescribe the pill more often than doctors at family planning clinics (83% and 59% respectively), who generally offer a wider range of contraceptive methods.[70]

Family planning clinics provide a range of specialist services, including psycho-social counselling; pregnancy testing; domiciliary family planning and special sessions for teenagers. A survey carried out by the Brook Advisory Centres in November 1995 found that 85–90% of health authorities provide special services for young people.

All family planning doctors and nurses working in clinics are required to have specialist qualifications in family planning. There is no requirement for postgraduate training among general practitioners or practice nurses. Patients of general practitioners are less likely to recall accurately secondary precautions necessary in the event of contraceptive failure.[71,30,32]

Abortion

Of conceptions in 1993, 80.8% led to maternities and 19.2% were terminated by abortion.[1]

ABORTION RATES

153 135 abortions were performed on women resident in England and Wales in 1995 (see Table 11).

Table 11 **Age-specific legal abortion rates per 1000 women: England and Wales 1995**

	Age	Total rate*
Under 16	3 240	5.22
16–19	24 724	21.59
20–24	43 077	24.38
25–29	36 986	18.10
30–34	25 592	12.63
35–39	14 228	8.07
40–44	4 831	2.86
45 and over	453	0.25
not stated	4	–
All ages	153 135	11.91

Source: ONS, 1996[2]

* Rates for 'all ages' are calculated on the basis of events at all ages (including those under 14 and over 49) in relation to the population of women who are aged 14–49. The rate (per 1000 women) for the under-16 age group is based on the population of women aged 14–15; for the 45 and over age group the rate is based on the population of women aged 45–49.

After a steady increase in the 1980s abortion rates have shown a decline in recent years (Figure 9). The 1995 figures show a 2.2% drop in numbers of abortions from the previous year, with the largest proportionate decrease of 4.0% among those aged 20–24.

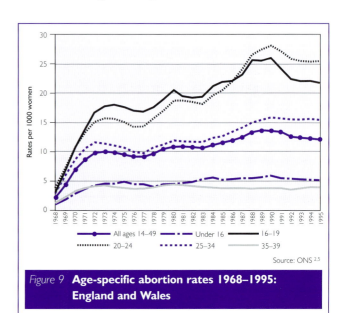

Source: ONS [2,5]

Figure 9 **Age-specific abortion rates 1968–1995: England and Wales**

Although conceptions and abortions among teenagers are a continual focus of attention, in recent years abortion rates among women in their early twenties have overtaken the rate for 16–19-year-olds. At 1991 rates 34.5 out of 100 women in England and Wales are expected to have at least one abortion during their reproductive lifetime, suggesting that unwanted pregnancy is a significant public health problem among women of all ages.

Factors influencing trends in legal abortions for residents of England and Wales include:

● Age of women – A changing age distribution of women within the 15–44 age range could have a profound effect on the overall number of terminations and the overall termination rate without changing the rates specific to each smaller age group within the 15–44 range. Around 6000 of the increase in number of terminations between 1980 and 1989 can be attributed to this factor.[4]

● Conception rates – A rise in conception rates (or increase in fertility) has in the past been reflected in higher abortion rates.[4]

● Attitudes/behaviour – Public concern with respect to more effective methods of contraception such as the pill coincided with a rise in abortion rates in the early 1980s.[5] Changing attitudes to abortion have made abortion a more acceptable choice[6] and the altered status and aspirations of women may also affect termination rates.[7]

● Service provision – The availability of services for abortion, family planning and emergency contraception.[5,8]

Parity
About half (53.1%) of abortions are among women with no children; 34.7% are performed for women with 1 or 2 children[2] and 66.3% are among single women.[9]

Socioeconomic group
Very little research has looked specifically at the association between social class and abortion; although a few studies have used other socioeconomic indicators in relation to teenage abortion rates.

A review of 8000 teenage pregnancies in Tayside, Scotland (1980–90) found that although there was a higher pregnancy rate in deprived areas of Tayside these

pregnancies were less likely to be terminated. Only 29.1% of pregnancies were terminated in the most deprived areas compared to 62.2% terminations in the most affluent areas.[10]

Ethnic group
Very little information is available on the frequency with which women from ethnic minorities seek termination. One survey of women seeking abortion in the Islington area found that 29.7% of the sample were black and 3% of Asian origin,[11] compared to 10.8% and 6% respectively of the whole female population of Islington.[12]

Region
Abortion rates vary within and between NHS regions. The highest numbers of abortions are among women 'usually resident' in the North Thames Region and the lowest in Anglia and Oxford Health Regions[2] (see Figure 10). Conversely, some of the lowest rates of abortions among under-16-year-olds are found in the Thames regions.[2]

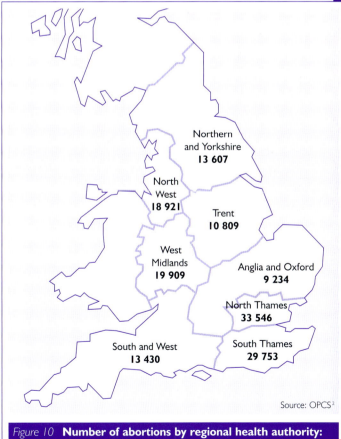

Source: OPCS[2]

Figure 10 **Number of abortions by regional health authority: England 1995**

International comparisons

Abortion rates vary considerably between European countries, reflecting both religious/socio-cultural differences and access to services (see Table 12). Generalisations are difficult to make, but low abortion rates have been associated with more open social acceptance of sexuality. This observation has been used to explain the dramatic differences in abortion rates between more sexually open Scandinavian societies and east European countries where abortion has been traditionally 'taboo' or recently illegal.

Table 12 **Number of abortions and abortion rate per 1000 women aged 15–44 by year: selected European countries and the United States**

Country and year	Abortions	Rate
Romania (1990)	914 000	183.6
Yugoslavia (1988)	343 300	66.7
Bulgaria (1988)	118 800	63.8
Czechoslovakia (1990)	157 300	45.7
China (1989)	10 379 400	37.5
Hungary (1994)	74 500	33.4
US (1992)	1 528 900	25.9
GDR (1988)	80 800	23.0
Singapore (1993)	16 500	22.7
Sweden (1994)	32 300	18.7
Denmark (1993)	18 700	16.9
Norway (1993)	14 900	16.1
Canada (1993)	104 400	15.3
England & Wales (1993)	157 800	14.7
Italy (1989)	171 700	13.5
France (1987)	161 000	13.3
Scotland (1993)	11 500	10.4
Finland (1993)	10 300	9.6
Switzerland (1984)	13 500	9.0
Spain (1987)	63 900	8.0
Netherlands (1994)	20 800	6.0
Ireland (1987)	3 700	4.8

Source: David[13] Henshaw[14] and Singh and Henshaw[15]

All figures obtained from official government services. Statistics based on survey data for Switzerland and Spain. Statistics are incomplete for France and Italy.

ABORTION AMONG TEENAGERS

Abortion rates among teenagers increased during the 1980s but have fallen since 1990.[9]

In 1993, 34.9% of all teenage conceptions led to a legal abortion, a slight increase on the preceding year (34.5%).

High teenage abortion rates in the UK compared to other European countries have been attributed partially to poor access to family planning services.[16]

In an exercise organised by the Brook Advisory Centres, a group of teenagers rang every fourth health authority on the NHS list to request either a prescription for the pill, free condoms or emergency contraception. Forty-four per cent of requests for help failed to get an appointment within a week and on 12% of occasions the teenagers were refused or put off by the attitude of the staff.[16] A local survey confirmed these findings.[17]

In a study of pregnant teenagers in Devon, those requesting abortion were younger and less likely to be in a stable relationship, and to have less contact with antenatal services than those who wanted to continue with the pregnancy.[18]

SERVICES

The three providers of abortion services in the UK are the National Health Service, charitable institutions and private clinics. In 1995, 70.4% of abortions in England and Wales were undertaken in NHS hospitals and/or undertaken in private clinics and paid for by the NHS while 29.6% of abortions were undertaken outside the NHS.[2]

In 1979 the Royal Commission on the NHS recommended that health authorities should aim to provide at least 75% of all abortions.[19]

Several studies show a consistent preference among women for NHS abortions but that many cite wanting a 'more sympathetic and faster service' as a reason for seeking private terminations.[20–22]

Evidence from one study showed that most patients (80%) request termination of pregnancy before 9 weeks of gestation; the mean delay between referral and operation was 20 days.[23] Despite this, 10.7% of women in England and Wales have abortions after the 12th week of pregnancy.[2] The rate of complications (such as infection, haemorrhage and damage to the uterus or cervix) is low but increases with gestational age (between 2 and 7 per 1000 depending on the method used and gestational age).[24]

Most abortions in the UK are performed as a surgical procedure.

RU486 (mifepristone), otherwise known as the 'abortion pill', has been found to be a safe and effective form of medical abortion.[25-27] Although originally restricted for use during the first 9 weeks of gestation, since July 1995 it has also been licensed for use between 13 and 20 weeks (it is not available for use between 9 and 13 weeks gestation due to side effects).

Faster referrals and more frequent use of RU486 could substantially reduce the complications rate, the distress for patients and staff associated with later abortions as well as saving NHS theatre time and financial resources.

Disadvantages of the abortion pill are that women experience some pain and bleeding, they have to make four or more visits to the hospital and are more likely to have an incomplete abortion than if they had had the foetus removed surgically.[14]

Suggestions for swifter referral systems include specialist abortion facilities, more cost-effectively staffed by junior doctors trained to perform abortions to which GPs can refer directly, and a centralised referral service. Trials of these systems in Edinburgh and Tower Hamlets have reduced late abortion rates by 50% to 75%.[28,29]

Acquired Immune Deficiency Syndrome (AIDS) and Human Immunodeficiency Virus (HIV)

AIDS (acquired immune deficiency syndrome) is a collection of specific illnesses and conditions that occur because the body's immune system has been damaged by the human immunodeficiency virus (HIV). HIV is transmitted via four main routes:

● through unprotected sexual intercourse (anal or vaginal)

● through the sharing of needles, hypodermic syringes or any other injecting equipment (injecting into veins, muscle or under skin)

● from an infected mother to her infant during pregnancy, birth or via breastfeeding

● by blood, either through infected blood factor or blood/tissue transfer (however, since 1985 all blood has been screened in the UK, blood products are treated[1] and this is no longer a main transmission route in the UK).

Certain other activities where blood or genital fluids could be exchanged may also carry some degree of risk; for example it is now thought that there is a risk of HIV transmission, although at extremely low rates, through oral sex.[2]

See Appendix 2 for background on the history and discovery of HIV and AIDS.

GLOBAL AND REGIONAL ESTIMATES OF AIDS AND HIV
Global context
The cumulative total number of adults and children *reported* to have AIDS throughout the world up to 30 June 1996 was 1 393 649, an increase of 19% from the 1 169 811 cases officially reported by 30 June 1995.[3] The number of reports of AIDS made to UNAIDS do not give an accurate global picture because reporting varies so much from one country to the next.

The joint United Nations Programme on HIV/AIDS provides estimates for AIDS and HIV on a global level, by different transmission categories.[4] Allowing for incomplete reporting, under-diagnosis, and reporting delay and based on available data on HIV infections around the world, the *estimated* true number of cumulative AIDS cases is 7.7 million since the epidemic began (Figure 11).

Since the beginning of the epidemic, it is estimated that more than 25.5 million adults have been infected with HIV and more than 4.5 million have died from HIV-related conditions. It is thought that there are currently 21.8 million people (800 000 children and 21 million adults) living with HIV/AIDS.[4]

Most cases occur amongst under-35s, and over 90% of deaths before the age of 49 years. Approximately 42% of adults living with HIV/AIDS are women, and this proportion is increasing.[4]

World-wide, unprotected heterosexual intercourse accounts for more than 70% of all adult HIV infections to date and intercourse between men for 5–10%. Transfusion of HIV-infected blood or blood products, on the other hand, accounts for 3–5% of all adult HIV infections. The sharing of HIV-infected injection equipment by drug users accounts for 5–10% of all adult HIV infections. This proportion is growing and in many areas of the world, injecting drug use is the dominant mode of transmission.[4]

Regional context

More than 90% of adults living with HIV or AIDS live in developing countries.[5] Table 13 shows the cumulative totals of AIDS reports and estimated AIDS cases, broken down by continent.

Table 13 **Cumulative AIDS cases by continent, up to 30 June 1996**

Continent	Number of AIDS reports	Estimates of AIDS cases (to nearest thousand)
Africa	501 714	5 929 000
Americas	181 174	462 000
(USA)	(411 907)	(539 000)
Asia	27 873	539 000
Europe	167 238	231 000
Oceania	*	*
World total	1 393 649	7 700 000

Source: UNAIDS[5]

* Less than 1%

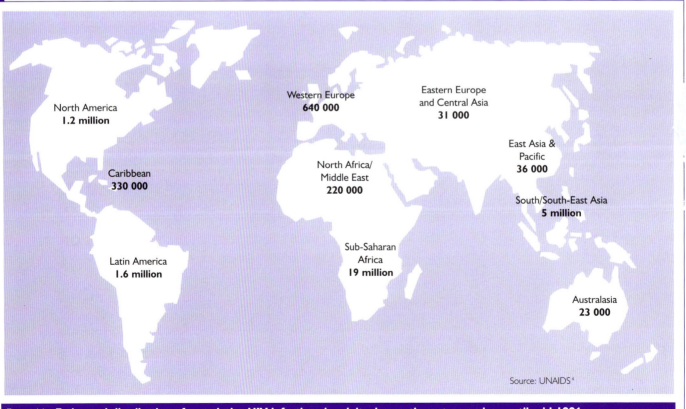

North America
1.2 million

Western Europe
640 000

Eastern Europe
and Central Asia
31 000

East Asia &
Pacific
36 000

Caribbean
330 000

North Africa/
Middle East
220 000

South/South-East Asia
5 million

Latin America
1.6 million

Sub-Saharan
Africa
19 million

Australasia
23 000

Source: UNAIDS[4]

Figure 11 **Estimated distribution of cumulative HIV infections in adults, by contingent or region, until mid-1996**

Europe

AIDS surveillance in Europe is carried out by the European Centre for the Epidemiological Monitoring of AIDS in France.[6] Figure 12 shows the incidence rate per million population of AIDS in 1995, for the 20 countries in Europe with the highest rates.

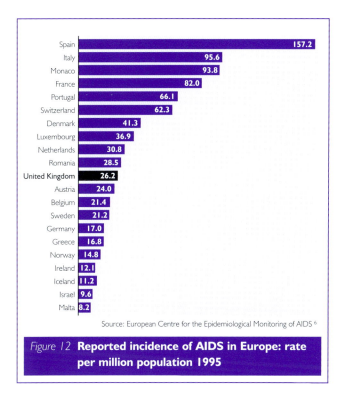

Source: European Centre for the Epidemiological Monitoring of AIDS [6]

Figure 12 **Reported incidence of AIDS in Europe: rate per million population 1995**

By this date a cumulative total of 171 811 AIDS cases had been reported in the 45 countries of the World Health Organization European region, with France, Italy and Spain accounting for 65% of all cases reported in Europe. The highest rates per million population in 1995 are reported in Spain (157.2), Italy (95.6), Monaco (93.8) and France (82.0). (The variations in reports between European countries may be influenced by different reporting procedures.)

The pattern of the epidemic varies within Europe; in most countries, including the UK, most people with HIV infection are gay or bisexual men. However, injecting drug users make up the largest group of people with AIDS in Ireland, Italy, Poland, Portugal, Spain and Ukraine. In Belgium, Bulgaria and Turkey the largest group of people with AIDS acquired the virus through heterosexual contact.[6]

AIDS AND HIV IN THE UNITED KINGDOM
Methods of surveillance

The AIDS Control Act (1987) requires health authorities and health boards to report each year the number of people with AIDS known to them. The main sources of

data come from the Public Health Laboratory Service's (PHLS) AIDS Centre at the Communicable Diseases Surveillance Centre (CDSC), the Scottish Centre for Infection and Environmental Health (SCIEH)[7] and the Institute of Child Health, London (ICH-L) in collaboration with CDSC and SCIEH. Appendix 3 provides an overview of the methods of data collection. These sources of data provide reports of HIV infection, AIDS cases, and AIDS deaths. In addition, the unlinked anonymous surveys monitor HIV prevalence among GUM and antenatal clinic attenders, injecting drug users, neonatal dried blood spots, hospital patients and pregnant women seeking terminations.

Prevalence and trends

The annual incidence of AIDS has risen almost six-fold between 1984 and 1994, with a steep rise in annual deaths between 1988 and 1993, though the death rate may now be stabilising.[8] The prevalence of AIDS cases in homosexual and bisexual males rose twelve-fold over the decade, reflecting high levels of HIV transmission early in the 1980s.[8]

The bulk of HIV transmission still occurs between men, with new reports rising in this category.[9,10] Transmission through heterosexual intercourse is increasing, and appears to be concentrated largely among those with partners from countries with high rates of heterosexual transmission and partners in 'high-risk' categories (injecting drug user, recipient of contaminated blood factor, bisexual man).[10] In recent years the number of infections reported from injecting drug users has remained more or less constant,[10] while the number of AIDS cases among children with infected mothers is rising.[8]

Figure 13 shows the overall trend in cumulative HIV infections up to 1995 by the main transmission categories.

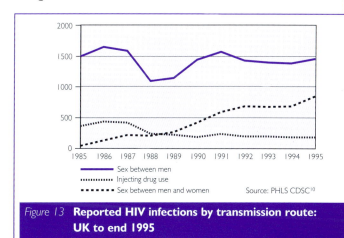

Source: PHLS CDSC[10]

Figure 13 **Reported HIV infections by transmission route: UK to end 1995**

As of the end of June 1996, there had been a cumulative total of 12 976 reports of people with AIDS and 9148 deaths from AIDS (Figure 14).[11] Figure 15 shows the trends in new cases of AIDS reported by year and the number of deaths between 1983 and 1995. In 1995, there were 1580 AIDS cases and 1219 deaths from AIDS.

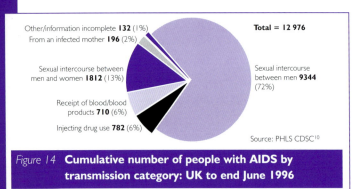

Figure 14 **Cumulative number of people with AIDS by transmission category: UK to end June 1996**

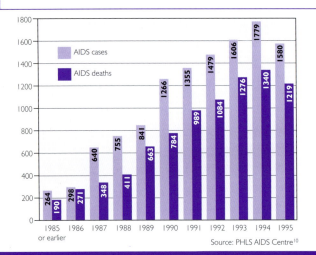

Figure 15 **New AIDS cases by year of report and deaths by year of known death: UK 1983–85**

By the end of June 1996 a *cumulative total* of 27 088 HIV reports (includes 55 of unknown sex) had been recorded in the UK (Figure 16).[11] In 1995 there were 2684 *new reports* of HIV.[10] Table 14 shows new cases by year and transmission category. New cases reflect the number of people being tested (for example, the high numbers in the early years reflect high uptake of the antibody test by certain groups, e.g. haemophiliacs, in the years immediately following the introduction of the test in 1984/85). Figure 17 shows in graphic form the trend in new reports.

Due to the time lapse between infection and development of AIDS, AIDS statistics should not be taken as representing transmission of HIV infection as it is today, but rather as it has occurred in the past (on average 10 years ago).

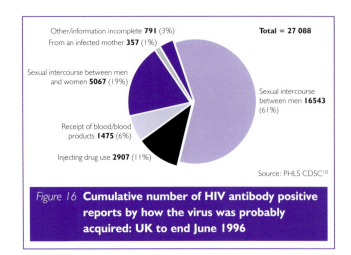

Figure 16 **Cumulative number of HIV antibody positive reports by how the virus was probably acquired: UK to end June 1996**

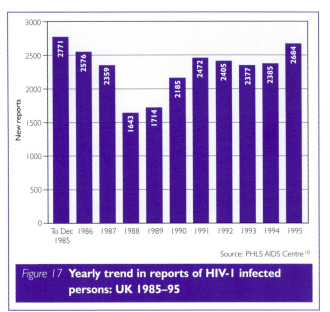

Figure 17 **Yearly trend in reports of HIV-1 infected persons: UK 1985–95**

Transmission categories
Sexual intercourse between men
Thus far cases of AIDS and deaths from AIDS have been concentrated among men who have sex with men. This category also continues to form the largest proportion of new AIDS cases reported each year (63.1% of new cases in 1995), although it has declined slightly (79.2% in 1989).[10]

As with AIDS, the majority of HIV is reported as transmitted through sexual intercourse between men, with 61.2% of cumulative reports to the end of June 1996 transmitted this way, compared to 18.7% through heterosexual sex.[10]

New reports of HIV infection among men who have sex with men increased in 1995, after a downward trend for the preceding three years. The Unlinked Anonymous HIV Prevalence Monitoring Programme concludes that 'the bulk of current HIV transmission is among homosexual and bisexual men and they remain the highest priority for preventive activities'.[9]

Table 14 **New cases of HIV-1 infection by transmission category: UK to the end of December 1995**

Year	Transmission category				
	Sexual intercourse between men	Sexual intercourse between men and women	Injecting drug use	Mother to infant	Blood and blood products
To end 1985	1 502	33	365	7	751
1986	1 628	115	431	11	317
1987	1 572	207	410	9	92
1988	1 096	199	228	11	44
1989	1 141	265	205	13	34
1990	1 444	413	189	31	64
1991	1 563	586	235	34	18
1992	1 437	667	195	54	25
1993	1 407	645	194	70	10
1994	1 400	667	185	65	22
1995	1 467	854	186	41	30

Source: PHLS AIDS Centre [10]

Because voluntary named testing can only pick up a proportion of people who are HIV positive, data from the programme of unlinked anonymous surveillance are valuable in estimating the proportion of the population with HIV.

As of 1994, the programme of unlinked anonymous surveillance estimated the following levels of HIV prevalence by category of sexual transmission.[9] In London and the south-east, at GUM clinics, prevalence of HIV was 11.33% (range 3.10–21.92%) of men with homosexual or bisexual exposure not known to have injected drugs.

Outside London and the south-east, numbers are much lower.[9] Again among GUM clinic attenders, it was estimated that 3.83% (range 1.40–4.50%) of homo/bisexually exposed men had HIV.

These data also facilitate predictions of the proportion of those with HIV who have not been diagnosed by voluntary named testing.[9] Data from GUM clinics suggest that in London and the south-east, 29% of homo/bisexual men with HIV have not been diagnosed. Outside London and the south-east, the figure is 34.9% of homosexual men with HIV.

Sexual intercourse between men and women
The proportion of new cases of AIDS contracted through sexual intercourse between men and women

has increased, from 8.3% of new cases in 1989 to 19.6% in 1995.[10]

Of the cumulative total of AIDS cases to end of June 1996, among those occurring through sex between men and women there were:

- 191 cases (10.5%) in which the partner was in a 'high-risk' category (i.e. injecting drug user, recipient of a blood transfusion or blood factor, bisexual man).

- 1420 cases (78.4%) in which the other partner came from, or had lived in countries where the major route of HIV-1 transmission is through sexual intercourse between men and women.

- 166 cases (9.2%) in which the sexual partner came from the UK and no high-risk activities were identified.

- 35 cases which are still under investigation.[10]

18.7% of cumulative reports of HIV to the end of June 1996 were transmitted through heterosexual sex.[10] HIV infections contracted from heterosexual intercourse generally continue to increase (see Figures 18 and 19), particularly in the last year, though numbers are relatively small.

Cumulative HIV reports to the end of June 1996 have broken down those cases transmitted by heterosexual intercourse as follows:

- 3763 (74%) reports from individuals with a sexual partner from abroad – this includes persons without other identified risks from, or who have lived in, countries where the major route of HIV-1 transmission is through sexual intercourse between men and women

- 601 (12%) reports from individuals with a 'high-risk' partner, i.e. a partner who is a bisexual male (this figure has remained low in both HIV and AIDS reports, suggesting that bisexuality has not been an important 'bridge' from gay men to women), an injecting drug user, a blood/components recipient or a haemophiliac

- 431 (9%) reports from those whose partner was from the UK and has no other obvious risk factor

- 272 (5%) in whom exposure category was undetermined.[11]

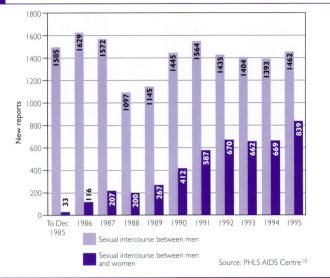

Figure 18 **Yearly trend in reports of HIV-1 infection contracted through sexual intercourse: UK 1985–95**

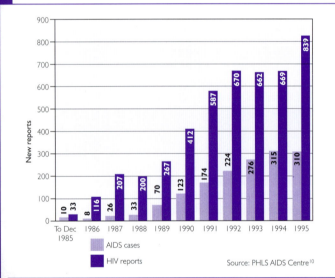

Figure 19 **Yearly trend in reports of HIV-1 infection and AIDS cases contracted through sexual intercourse between men and women: UK 1985–95**

Again the unlinked anonymous surveillance programme provides further insight into estimated levels of HIV infection.

As of 1994, it was estimated that in London and the south-east, at GUM clinics, prevalence of HIV was 0.90% (range 0.31–2.12%) of men with heterosexual exposure and 0.48% of heterosexual women (range 0.12–0.80%).

Among GUM clinic attenders outside London and the south-east, it was estimated that 0.14% (range 0.0–0.36%) of heterosexually exposed men had HIV, and 0.04% (range 0.0–0.14%) of heterosexually exposed women.

Data from GUM clinics also suggest that in London and the south-east, 69.9% of heterosexual men and 50% of heterosexual women with HIV have not been diagnosed. Outside London and the south-east, the figures are 71.8% of heterosexual men and 55.6% of heterosexual women with HIV.

The unlinked anonymous survey reports that a large proportion of heterosexual HIV transmission reports have been among people who either spent time, or had intercourse with someone who spent time, abroad in high HIV prevalence countries, mainly Sub-Saharan Africa. In 1994, 81% (390 of 479) of all heterosexually transmitted reported cases of HIV were believed to have been acquired through an association with time spent abroad.[9]

Intravenous drug use

The United Kingdom has a relatively low number of drug users among the total cases of AIDS (6.1%) compared with countries such as Italy and Spain where, by June 1996, about two-thirds of total AIDS cases were in this group.[6] A total of 550 men and 232 women had developed AIDS following HIV infection via injecting drug use, of whom 529 had died. A further 224 were men who had had sex with men.[11] In 1994 there were 24 703 drug misusers (the majority non-injecting) notified to the Home Office.[12] However it has been estimated that there may be 75 000–150 000 drug users in the United Kingdom, of whom approximately 50% may be injecting drug users.[13]

Statistics to the end of June 1996 indicate that a cumulative total of 2903 people have become infected with HIV-1 through injecting drug use.[11] A further 339 cases were in injecting drug users who are also homosexual or bisexual men. Of these cases, 1076 (37.4%) were reported in Scotland and 1194 (41.5%) were reported in North Thames and South Thames regions.[10] Figure 20 shows that in recent years the number of infections reported from injecting drug users has remained more or less constant.

Data from the unlinked anonymous surveys estimate HIV prevalence among injecting drug users attending specialist agencies at 3.0% (0.30–0.94%) of men, and 4.0% (1.6–7.4%) of women. Outside the south-east, these are 0.3% (0.0–0.7%) of men and 0.6% (0.0–3.7%) of women.[9]

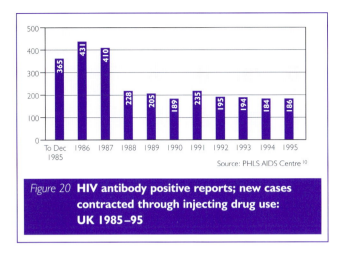

Source: PHLS AIDS Centre [10]

Figure 20 HIV antibody positive reports; new cases contracted through injecting drug use: UK 1985–95

Through blood products

Of new AIDS cases in 1995, 7.0% were contracted though blood transfer or factor, compared with 6.2% in 1989.[10]

Of those in the PHLS statistics of HIV reports who were assumed to have contracted HIV via blood, blood product or tissue transfer (5.3% of cumulative total), the majority (87.1%) had contracted it through an infected blood product (e.g. haemophiliacs), while the rest (12.9%) contracted it through blood or tissue transfer (e.g. through transfusion or transplantation).[11]

Mother to child

As Table 14 shows, there is also an upward trend among children who have contracted HIV from their mothers. Though numbers here are still very small, this group is rising most quickly (the fall in 1995 is an artefact that occurs every year due to time lags in reporting).

Data from the unlinked anonymous surveys indicate that 0.171% of pregnant women at delivery were HIV positive in London and the south-east, and 0.010% outside this region. Of women seeking termination of pregnancy, 0.62% had HIV in London and the south-east.[9]

In addition, of pregnant women with HIV, it is estimated that 83% of those in London and the south-east, and 90% of those in the rest of England and Wales have not been diagnosed through voluntary testing.[9] The Unlinked Anonymous HIV Prevalence Monitoring Programme concludes that these proportions are disturbingly high given the availability of ways of reducing the risk of mother-to-child transmission.[9]

Variations

Sex

At the end of June 1996 there was a cumulative total of 11 708 cases of AIDS among men and 1268 among women; 8419 men and 729 women had died from AIDS.[11]

So far, because the main mode of transmission to date has been sexual intercourse between men, HIV and AIDS have affected men more than women (at a ratio of roughly 6:1 for HIV). However, the proportion of new reports of HIV among women has increased gradually. For instance, in 1989 12.5% of new reports where the sex was known were in women. In 1995 this had increased to 20.5%.[10]

For women, heterosexual sex is the most significant transmission category, at 65.9% of total HIV cases.[11] Most of these infections occurred outside the UK or were in women who had sex with high-risk partners (i.e. injecting drug users, haemophiliacs or men who had sex with men).

Age group

Thus far, the HIV epidemic has been concentrated in young adults. This is likely to be because of the nature of the major routes of transmission – unprotected sex with one or more partners and injecting drug use – practices which are more common among younger adults. Reports of HIV infections tend to be concentrated in the age range of 20–39. This has not changed significantly in recent years.[10]

At the end of June 1996, 58.0% of males and 65.9% of females who have developed AIDS were in the age group 25–39. Proportionally women with AIDS are more likely to be younger than men with AIDS; 18.4% of cases among women are in under-25s, compared with only 5.2% of cases among men.[10] The same applies for HIV infection; 32.2% of infections among women and 17.7% of infections among men are under 25 years of age.

Children (14 or under at diagnosis). A total of 247 AIDS cases in children aged 14 years or less at diagnosis was reported by the end of April 1996, 130 of whom are known to have died; 195 (78.9%) were vertically infected (i.e. transmission from mother to child before or during birth or through breastfeeding) and 51 (20.6%) were infected through contaminated blood or blood factor treatment.[11]

In this time period, there were also 669 reports of children with HIV. Though numbers are small, this group is rising most quickly. The majority of cases in this age group occur among African females (see Table 16) and in the London region.

Table 15 **Age distribution of HIV-1 infected persons:
UK cumulative totals to end June 1996**

Age group (years when diagnosed)	Reports of HIV-1			
	Male	Female	Total*	%
0–4	185	158	345	1
5–14	281	41	324	2
15–19	549	167	718	3
20–24	2 990	913	3 909	15
25–29	5 303	1 209	6 518	24
30–34	4 852	830	5 687	21
35–39	3 457	329	3 788	14
40–44	2 208	146	2 356	9
45–49	1 315	66	1 381	5
50–54	759	54	813	3
55+	761	65	827	3
Total	**22 660**	**3 987**	**26 666**	**100**
Age unknown	341	54	422	

Source: PHLS AIDS Centre[10]
* includes 55 for whom sex is not noted

By the end of April 1996, of 886 children born to mothers with HIV since 1979 in the UK, 357 are now known to be infected, 271 uninfected, and the remaining 258 undetermined.[11] A child born to an HIV positive mother will only be recorded as being HIV positive if the virus has been isolated, antibody to HIV persists after 18 months, or if there has been progression to AIDS.[11]

Neonates (babies up to 4 weeks old). All babies born to HIV positive mothers initially carry HIV antibody. Infection status among mothers is tested by sampling dried blood spots from neonates (who still possess maternal antibodies). In 1994, the unlinked anonymous survey of dried blood spots showed HIV prevalence in London to be approximately 28 times the rate outside London (0.28% for those resident in inner London and 0.01% for those resident outside London).[9]

Ethnic group
Statistics for HIV infection are not collected by ethnic group, but ethnic group information is available for 89% of AIDS reports. Table 16 summarises the ethnic group of AIDS cases reported to the end of June 1996.

Though overall the majority of AIDS cases are among men who have sex with men, this is not the case for all ethnic groups. Among those in the 'black' category, 70.5% of people with AIDS contracted HIV through

Table 16 **Ethnic group of reported AIDS cases:
UK cumulative totals to end June 1996**

Exposure category	White	Black	Asian or Oriental	Other or mixed	Total
Sexual intercourse between men	8 084	221	109	174	9 344
Sexual intercourse between men and women	575	935	69	46	1 812
Injecting drug use	585	14	1	3	782
Blood	420	14	22	19	710
Mother to infant	37	129	3	22	196
Other/ undetermined	97	13	4	3	132
Total	**9 798**	**1 326**	**208**	**267**	**12 976**

The table excludes a breakdown of those cases where ethnic group is not known, but these cases are included in the last column.
Source: PHLS CDSC[10]

heterosexual intercourse, and just 16.7% through sex between men. Sex between men accounts for just over half (52.4%) of AIDS cases among 'Asian or Oriental' people, and, following the national trend, of 82.5% of people in the 'white' ethnic category. It should be noted that among certain ethnic groups, such as Asian and Oriental, numbers are still very small.

There is a consensus that the epidemic in the UK is fuelled mainly by the course of the epidemic in Africa laid over existing infection trends.[9]

Region
The majority of AIDS cases (63.2%) in the UK are concentrated in the two Thames regions. Deaths follow a similar pattern.[10] This proportion has changed little since reporting began in the 1980s.

The majority of reports of HIV infected persons are also located in a few regions (Figure 21), though reports have been made from all regions in the UK.

The authors of the 1995 report from unlinked anonymous surveillance concluded that the data confirmed London is the focus of the HIV epidemic in

England, and that the extent to which the epidemic is affecting women in London, especially younger women, is worrying (it is estimated that 1900 women aged 20–34 in London may be HIV positive).

PROJECTIONS

There have been a number of projections of the way that the HIV epidemic will spread in England and Wales, including the Cox Report[14] in 1988 and the Day Reports.[15,16,8]

The Day Reports predict, for planning purposes, the actual number of people with HIV and AIDS in the UK (as opposed to the number known) and the pattern of the epidemic in the future.

The 1996 Day Report[8] estimates that at the end of 1993 there were 21 900 (range 20 400 to 23 400) HIV-infected adults (living) in the population compared with 10 680 reported HIV-infected adults alive for the same period. Thus almost 49% of adults living with HIV may not have been identified.

Of these 21 900 estimated cases:

● 12 350 (56.4%) will have been infected through sex between men. There were actually 6865 reports, suggesting 44.4% were unaware of their HIV positive status.

● 2050 (9.4%) through injecting drug use, compared with 1170 reports – 42.9% may have been unaware of their status.

● 6800 (31.1%) through sex between men and women, compared with only 2235 reports – suggesting 67.1% of people who contracted HIV heterosexually were unaware of the fact.

● 700 (3.2%) blood or blood factor recipients, compared with 410 reports – suggesting 41.4% may be unaware.

Data from unlinked anonymous screening programmes and from the National Survey of Sexual Attitudes and Lifestyles (NASSAL)[17] played an important part in the calculations made of the numbers of HIV-infected people in England and Wales in 1993. The report is based on AIDS case reports to the end of December 1994.

For those implementing local and national prevention initiatives the results indicate the need for sustained

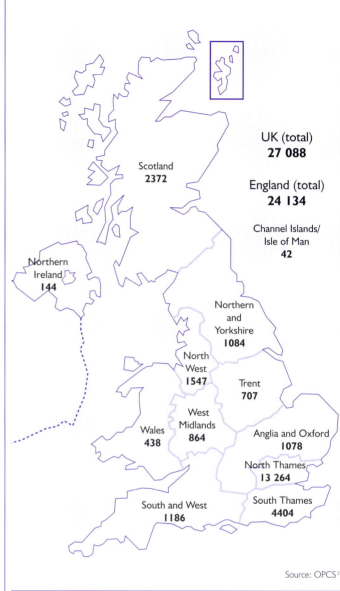

UK (total)
27 088

England (total)
24 134

Channel Islands/
Isle of Man
42

Scotland
2372

Northern
Ireland
144

Northern
and
Yorkshire
1084

North
West
1547

Trent
707

West
Midlands
864

Wales
438

Anglia and Oxford
1078

North Thames
13 264

South and West
1186

South Thames
4404

Source: OPCS[2]

Figure 21   **Geographical distribution of HIV-1 reports (cumulative) as at March 1996**

prevention efforts to be directed at homo/bisexual men, heterosexuals at risk of other STDs, and IDUs. The numbers of undiagnosed cases suggest that prevention and HIV testing need to be carefully targeted.[9]

Table 17 summarises the planning projections for 1997 and 1999 for the incidence of AIDS among the main exposure categories, adjusting for underreporting (i.e. number of new cases per year).

At the end of 1999, it is projected that there will be about 4000 people with AIDS alive in the population (England and Wales) and about 4000 people with severe HIV infection.

It is predicted that AIDS incidence will begin to level off in 1997 and 1999 (Figure 22).

Table 17 **Estimated new cases of AIDS in 1997 and 1999 by transmission category, including upper and lower limits of estimates for total AIDS cases, England and Wales**

1997	Lower	Upper	Planning
AIDS cases	1 840	2 300	2 025
Homosexual and bisexual men	985	1 360	1305
IDUs	95	155	140
Heterosexual men and women	365	495	490

1999	Lower	upper	Planning
AIDS cases	1 760	2 455	2010
Homosexual and bisexual men	865	1 445	1235
IDUs	105	180	155
Heterosexual men and women	390	540	525

Source: PHLS CDSC[8]

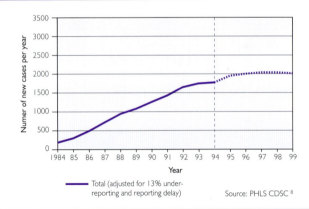

Total (adjusted for 13% under-reporting and reporting delay)

Source: PHLS CDSC [8]

Figure 22 **Observed (1984–94) and projected (1995–99) annual incidence of AIDS using data to end June 1994: England and Wales**

Modes of transmission

Although data suggest that HIV transmission among men who have sex with men or men who are bisexual declined markedly between 1983 and 1987, there are indications that HIV transmission probably increased again from 1989 onwards.[8]

Compared with the 1993 report, the planning projection for AIDS incidence among men who have sex with men in 1997 has fallen by 3% because the

1993 report presented an over-optimistic view of the extent to which patients receive treatment and prophylaxis before the onset of AIDS.[8]

The planning projections for 1997 are 37% lower for cases acquired heterosexually, resulting from the substantial decline in the rate of increase in the number of new AIDS cases arising each year from heterosexual exposure.[8]

The number of annual deaths from AIDS is projected to rise from 1145 in 1994 to over 2000 in 1999.[8]

A report from the University of Birmingham which uses a computer simulation model to predict the future incidence and prevalence of HIV infections suggested that the one single factor that could most influence the spread of the epidemic among heterosexuals is condom use rather than, for example, frequency of partner change.[18]

It is still difficult to predict the course of the epidemic with certainty. The findings of the 1996 Day Report depend on a number of assumptions and will be affected by the following factors:

● if indications of a recent increase in transmission among homosexual/bisexual men continue;

● by sexual mixing among subsets of the heterosexual population about which little is known;

● if needle-sharing behaviour changes;

● if future survival and treatment effects alter.

Scotland

A report of a working group convened by the Chief Medical Officer for Scotland (December 1995) predicted the number of AIDS cases and severe HIV-related disease for Scotland to the end of 1999.[19]

It is predicted that the number of new AIDS cases will increase by 10% from 140 in 1995 to 155 in 1999.[19]

The number of people living with AIDS is expected to increase by approximately 12% over the same period from 240 to 270.[19]

The number of people with severe HIV-related disease, including AIDS, is expected to increase by a similar percentage from 545 in 1995 to 610 in 1999.[19]

These trends are due to predicted large increases in cases among heterosexual men and women; little change in the numbers of cases among injecting drug users and homosexual/bisexual men is expected.[19]

THE ECONOMIC COSTS OF AIDS AND HIV

For an individual in England, from the time of infection, the cost of care for a lifetime has been estimated at £80 239.[20] This could represent a figure of about £133 million per year (if 'lifetime' is taken to be 10 years from the time of diagnosis, and taking the number of people known to have HIV or AIDS in 1995). Other estimates of costs incurred by the NHS in treating HIV and AIDS are at around a minimum of £1.65 billion.[21]

These figures relate to care and do not include the cost of drugs. The cost of AZT per year could add another £8 million.[20] Clinical trials of a new multiple-drug therapy have been carried out, which is expected to cost over $10 000 for one year's course of therapy for one person.[22]

The burden in terms of mortality associated with AIDS marks out HIV from the other areas of sexual health. From a financial point of view this has serious implications with respect to working years and life years lost.

AIDS has become one of the leading causes of death in younger people in some parts of the world. In the United States it is the second commonest cause of death in men aged 25–44. In the UK London is hardest hit. HIV was found to be the leading cause of death in male residents aged 15–44 of Riverside district health authority in London.[23]

By 1989 it was calculated that total life years lost from AIDS in the UK was 0.73% of the total from all causes, and working years lost came to over 4% of the total.[24]

Government spending

By 1993 it was estimated that the British government had devoted £1 billion towards HIV and AIDS. The cumulative government spending on research related to HIV and AIDS to the end of March 1994 was £130 million. The largest amount of funding is via the Medical Research Council.[25]

Billions of dollars worldwide are invested in research into HIV and AIDS, and between 1981 and 1992 36 000 papers on AIDS had been published in the major scientific journals.[26]

Relatively small amounts are spent on health education related to HIV and AIDS. In the financial year 1992/93 nearly £4 million was spent on mass media advertising by the Health Education Authority. At the end of the 1980s media advertising was at its peak and spending on advertising by the condom industry was over £1 million a year.[27]

KNOWLEDGE OF AND BELIEFS ABOUT AIDS AND HIV

Results from an HEA tracking survey among people in the United Kingdom aged 13+ indicate that great strides forward have been made in terms of knowledge of HIV. When asked to name the virus which causes AIDS, only 24% of respondents in 1988 knew that it was HIV. When prompted, an additional 58% recognised the term HIV, a total of 82% total awareness. However, in 1991, this had increased to 97% total awareness.[28] Figure 23 shows this trend. Data from 1993 (unpublished) indicate that 85% of adults aged 16–54 are able to name the virus causing AIDS without prompting.[29]

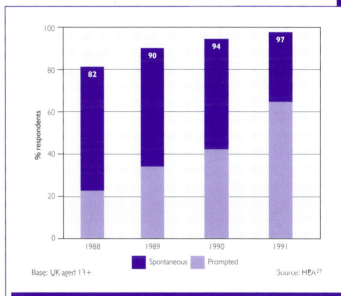

Base: UK aged 13+   Source: HEA[29]

Figure 23 **Spontaneous and prompted recognition of HIV as the virus which causes AIDS: UK 1988–1991**

Over this time period, there has been a growing certainty that 'most' or all people with HIV are likely to develop AIDS. The factors which contribute to the speed that this might happen remain, however, not fully understood. Most people experience 8 to 10 years without any major symptoms.

Figure 24 shows the percentage of respondents who believe that HIV can be transmitted via particular routes.[30]

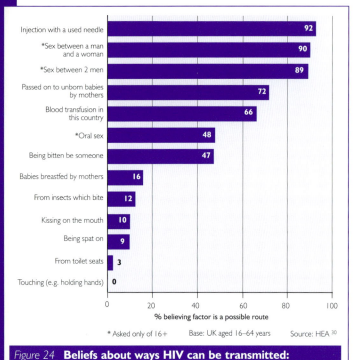

Figure 24   Beliefs about ways HIV can be transmitted: UK 1996

In 1992, 34% of women and 42% of men (aged 16–54) felt very well informed about the risks of HIV/AIDS. Another 43% of women and 45% of men felt fairly well informed.[31] There is thus a substantial proportion of the population who feel that they understand the risks of HIV.

ATTITUDES

Attitudes towards people with HIV and AIDS

Statistics from HEA surveys indicate that the majority of adults have a sympathetic attitude towards those people who are infected with HIV or have AIDS. Latest available statistics from 1991 among people in the UK aged 13+ show that:

● 31% feel that anyone who catches HIV (the AIDS virus) has only themselves to blame.

● 18% believe that people with HIV (the AIDS virus) should be put into quarantine to keep them away from the public (this declined from 24% in 1989).

● 76% believe that people with AIDS should be allowed to live in the community normally.[28]

There is some evidence that there has been a continuing growth in sympathy towards people with HIV and AIDS since tracking began in 1988. However, it should be noted that in the face of reality, even of distant personal relevance, 'theoretical sympathy' can dissolve rapidly.[28]

Sexually transmitted diseases other than HIV infection

INTRODUCTION

Sexually transmitted diseases (STDs) other than HIV infection are themselves a major cause of ill health, and can have long-term consequences such as infertility, ectopic pregnancy, chronic pelvic pain and genital cancers. The main burden of the sequelae of infections falls upon women. STDs are often asymptomatic, for example, gonorrhoea and chlamydial infection can lead to pelvic inflammatory disease (PID), which is also mostly asymptomatic, yet can cause infertility.[1] A rise in the incidence of chlamydia in the 1980s was matched by a rise in hospital admissions for PID. Registrations of cervical cancer increased at a time when attendance at GUM clinics for genital warts was also increasing.[2]

Cure of most STDs is relatively inexpensive and simple, if detected and treated early. Although very little work has been done to determine the costs to the NHS of STDs, total costs of diseases of the genitourinary system were estimated at £874 million in 1994 for the UK. This excludes the costs of some of the more serious sequelae of some STDs such as infertility or cervical cancer.[3]

(See Appendix 4 for definitions of STDs and their symptoms.)

SOURCES OF INFORMATION

Evidence from developing countries in particular suggests that other sexually transmitted diseases, present in people with HIV, may facilitate the transmission of HIV infection.[4,5]

The most consistent and comprehensive sources of data on STDs in England are the genito-urinary medicine (GUM) clinic returns to the Public Health Laboratory Service Communicable Disease Surveillance Centre (before July 1996, these were made to the Department of Health). Each NHS GUM clinic in England makes these returns quarterly. See Table 18 (returns from clinics in Wales, Northern Ireland and Scotland are made to their respective Health Departments).

GUM clinic returns report on the number of new attendances for specific conditions (as well as visits by

Table 18 **Number of new cases seen at GUM[†] clinics: England 1995**

Wart virus	93 317
Candidiasis*	69 432
Chlamydia	39 289
Herpes	27 065
Gonorrhoea	12 359
Trichomoniasis	5 486
Pediculosis and scabies	5 478
Syphilis	1 417

* Not necessarily sexually acquired
† These are now often referred to as sexual health clinics
Source: Department of Health [6]

those who do not require treatment). The figures are indicators of the incidence of STDs in England, though many STDs will be treated by GPs and therefore not necessarily shown in statistics. The total number of cases shown does not reflect the total number of patients; for example, a patient may attend once with more than one condition, in which case each is counted, or the same patient may re-attend a number of times a year with a new condition and will be classified as a case for each re-infection or recurrence.

GUM clinic data are thought to under-report incidence among adolescents and possibly women, who are more likely to attend other clinics or GPs for treatment. Also it is known that some important STDs are frequently asymptomatic, especially in women. Examples are gonorrhoea, chlamydia infection and HIV.

Changes in the classification of data on the GUM returns in 1988 require that caution is applied in interpreting trend data between 1980 and 1990. Chlamydia, for example, was not classified separately from all non-specific genitourinary infection (NSGI) until 1988.*

Complete data on pelvic inflammatory disease (PID) (a consequence of some gonorrhoea and chlamydia infections) are not available from GUM clinic returns, and most information on this disease comes from hospital discharge data.

* Testing for chlamydia was not widely available before 1988. It is still not necessarily used in all clinics and testing procedures also vary. The overall total for non-specific urethritis (NSU) and chlamydia should, however, be an accurate indication of trends.

TRENDS

New attendances at GUM clinics rose significantly in the mid-1980s (with a fall in cases of acute STD between 1986 and 1988). Since 1989 attendances with new conditions have been increasing by 1–2% per year with greater increases between 1993 and 1995. The total number of new cases seen at GUM clinics in 1995 was 404 638, an increase of approximately 6% over 1994 (excluding HIV/AIDS). The number of new cases in males rose by 4% and females by 8%; 176 423 were men and 228 215 were women.[6]

Trends over time will also reflect improvements or changes in diagnostic techniques and clinic organisation.

There was a decline in the incidence of gonorrhoea and syphilis during the 1980s but rises in the incidence of herpes, genital warts, and candidiasis (three of the most common STDs seen at GUM clinics).[6]

Trends for the more common conditions are shown in Figure 25.

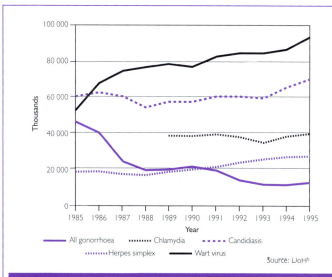

Figure 25 **New cases of selected conditions: England 1985–95**

Gonorrhoea

The *Health of the Nation* target for gonorrhoea has now been surpassed.[6] In 1995 there were 12 359 new cases identified in GUM clinics in England, 5% higher than 1994.

There were dramatic rises in the incidence of gonorrhoea among both sexes in the period following the Second World War and again in the 1960s. After a period throughout the 1970s and early 1980s when the annual number of cases was 50 000 or more, the number fell rapidly to 20 000 by 1988. According to the Department of Health's annual report on new cases, this drop was probably a result of safer sex campaigns introduced to prevent the spread of HIV. This level was maintained until 1991, but successive falls of 24%, 17% and 2% in the years to 1994 brought the annual total to just under 12 000. Thereafter, incidence started rising in mid- to late 1994.[6]

This upward trend appears to be accounted for mainly by an increase in the rate among males in the 25–34-year-old age group. Of new cases in men, the proportion which were reported as acquired through homosexual contact (estimated at 23%) may be increasing.[6]

Chlamydia

The annual number of new cases of *chlamydia trachomatis* identified in GUM clinics has remained at between 33 000 and 38 000 since 1989. However, the number of cases rose by 15.6% between 1993 and 1995 to 39 289, the highest since 1989. In 1995 the rise was 7%, greater than that for any other sexually transmitted disease.

These are likely to be underestimates; there may be many cases not recorded in these statistics because they have been identified in places other than GUM clinics.[6]

New cases in men accounted for 46% of the total in 1996, compared with 44% in 1989. Of cases in men, only a very small proportion (1.9%) were reported as acquired through sex between men.

Recently the concern about and media attention to chlamydia has grown in strength, particularly because of its potential for causing pelvic infection and infertility in women. In addition, changes in the methods of testing for the disease over the past five years have led to their wider use and increased sensitivity, allowing general practitioners to identify the many previously undetected asymptomatic cases.[7]

The Department of Health established in 1996 an Expert Advisory Group on *Chlamydia trachomatis* to advise the Chief Medical Officer and Ministers on screening for the disease and monitoring its sequelae. A report is expected later in 1997 with recommendations for effective action.

Herpes

The number of cases has been steadily increasing since 1988, when the total was under 17 000. In 1995, the total was 27 065, an increase of 1% over 1994 figures, though this included recurrence attacks (44% of the total).[6]

The number of first attacks fell by 2% in 1995, the first annual fall since 1989 when such cases were reported separately. The number of cases in males fell by 6% but in females rose slightly, accounting for 61% of all first attacks.[6]

Wart virus

The number of cases of genital warts was 93 317, an increase of 8% over the total for 1994. Recurrence attacks and re-registered cases accounted for 45% of the total in 1995, the number of first attacks being an increase of 5% over 1994 at 51 260. First attacks among females accounted for 49% of the total in 1995. Of the new cases in men about 5% were reported as being acquired through sex between men.[6]

VARIATIONS
Sex

Female cases of herpes outnumbered male cases in 1993 and 1994 as did chlamydia. The great majority of cases of candidiasis and trichomoniasis are seen in women.

Increases in viral and chlamydial infection among women in the 1980s are of concern because of the serious sequelae of these conditions. A rise in incidence of chlamydia in the 1980s was paralleled by a rise in hospital admissions for PID. It was noted that registrations of cervical cancer increased at a time when attendance at GUM clinics for genital warts was also increasing.[2]

Figure 26 shows the distribution of cases between men and women.

Age

Adolescents are less likely to be referred to GUM clinics, which may lead to an underestimate of incidence in this age group and an overestimate of the mean age of infection. A study of 121 teenage clinic attenders found that rates of most STDs were higher than the national average; females were found to have a high prevalence of genital warts.[8]

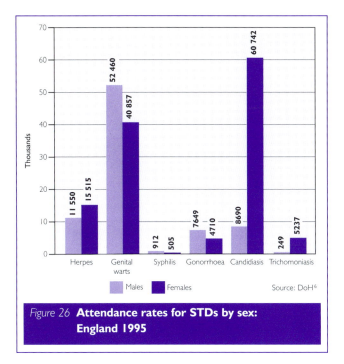

Figure 26 **Attendance rates for STDs by sex: England 1995**

The fall in incidence of gonorrhoea during the 1980s occurred primarily amongst over-25-year-olds,[2] which could suggest that younger people are less likely to take precautionary measures against STDs; the highest rates in women occurred at 16–19 years and in men at 20–24 years; this could reflect a higher number of sexual partners in this age group.

In 1995, rates were highest in women aged 20–24 years and for men aged 25–34 years.[9]

Figure 27 shows the median age of GUM clinic attenders by condition.

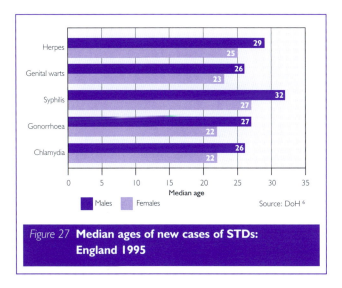

Figure 27 **Median ages of new cases of STDs: England 1995**

Sexual orientation
Homosexually acquired gonorrhoea fell between 1980 and 1988 suggesting a trend toward safer sex among sexually active homosexual men.[2,10]

However, a prospective study of a large cohort of 691 men recruited from the gay community in 1988/89 found that an increasing proportion were reporting anal intercourse and that the numbers of partners were increasing.[11] The study predicted a subsequent rise in HIV and rectal gonorrhoea. Although GUM clinic data for homosexually acquired cases are incomplete,[12] a number of studies have shown a rise in incidence among this group.[6,13–15] Overall, laboratory reports of rectal gonorrhoea in England and Wales increased fourfold between 1989 and 1990.[2] In 1995, 23.2% of new cases of gonorrhoea in men were reported as acquired through sex with other men.[6]

It has been argued that an upturn in gonorrhoea among gay and bisexual men reflects an increase in 'risky' sexual activity within an active core group, rather than a reversal in the overall trend toward safer sex among all homosexual men.[16] However, the distinction between 'core' and 'non-core' groups is not clear cut, and not enough is known about how these groups mix. Meanwhile there is evidence for the need to continue to target health education messages towards younger men who have become sexually active since the awareness of HIV and AIDS peaked in the mid-1980s .[17]

Increases in cases of chlamydia, genital herpes and warts among heterosexuals are suggested by trends seen for females.[2]

AWARENESS AND ATTITUDES
Responses from 838 adults aged 16–64 interviewed during 1996 for the Health Education Authority showed that public understanding of STDs is poor.[18]

Gonorrhoea was the most well-known STD (84% of respondents said they had heard of it) but only 69% had heard of genital warts, and 28% had heard of chlamydia.

Women were better informed about STDs than men but not in the case of gonorrhoea.

UPTAKE OF SERVICES
The Health of the Nation states that development of sexual health services, and the establishment of easily accessible service provision for the residents of every district, should continue to be a priority within the NHS.[19]

Attendance rates in some parts of the country are much higher than in other parts,[20] reflecting both variations in the incidence of STDs and the accessibility and availability of services.

One quarter's figures of GUM clinic attendances show attendance rates for the former North East Thames, North West Thames and south-east Thames regions to be double or more than double rates for other regions in England. The West Midlands had the lowest rate of attendance.[20]

Lower rates of STDs reported from GUM clinics in rural areas may reflect lower rates of infection in these areas or may reflect the greater use made in such areas of general practitioner services, as well as the fact that people may travel to cities for treatment.

STDs AS SENTINEL INDICATORS

Trends in STD incidence are frequently cited as sentinel or proxy indicators of sexual behaviour and/or of rates of HIV transmission.[14,21,22] A study in a London GUM clinic between 1985 and 1991 found that people with HIV were three times more likely to have had another STD than controls matched for sex, sexual orientation, injecting drug use and age at the time of the test.[23] For this reason, the reduction of gonorrhoea was chosen as a *Health of the Nation* target.[19] Due to difficulties inherent in the HIV and AIDS statistics, no specific *Health of the Nation* target for HIV has been possible. While there are good reasons to use this approach, a number of important factors make gonorrhoea and other STDs imperfect indicators of sexual behaviour and HIV transmission.

Health of the Nation Target

To reduce the incidence of gonorrhoea among men and women aged 15–64 by at least 20% by 1995 (from 61 new cases per 100 000 population in 1990 to no more than 49 cases per 100 000).

Objectives

To reduce the incidence of other sexually transmitted diseases.

● To develop further and strengthen monitoring and surveillance.

● To provide effective services for the diagnosis and treatment of STDs.

Sexual behaviour

Gonorrhoea has been used to indicate trends in sexual behaviour because it was endemic (habitually present in the community), relatively common, with a short incubation period, and people remain susceptible to gonorrhoea even after they have been treated (unlike other infectious diseases), so there was not a significant population with immunity to gonorrhoea. Although a number of other factors* may affect the trend in the incidence of gonorrhoea and other STDs in general, gonorrhoea is considered a reasonably reliable indicator of sexual behaviour.[21,24–26]

As gonorrhoea becomes increasingly uncommon, however, it will become a less reliable indicator of sexual behaviour: those practising higher-risk behaviours are less likely to encounter gonorrhoea, and in some areas of the country it may not be found at all.

HIV transmission

The unlinked anonymous HIV prevalence monitoring programme has shown that risk of acquiring another sexually transmitted disease continues to be a powerful predictor of risk for HIV infection in heterosexual men and women.[27] However, they are not completely reliable indicators for a number of reasons.

The spread of HIV in the population differs from diseases which have been endemic for some time. Secondly, people with HIV, unlike people with other STDs, have periods when they are more infectious than at other times, which can account for its rapid spread when first introduced into a highly sexually active population (for example among gay men in San Francisco).[28]

Moreover, the relationship between specific behaviours and transmission is still poorly understood. A change in behavioural factors which may reduce the incidence of gonorrhoea for example, will not necessarily lead to a reduction in the rate of HIV in the population.[29,30]

Hepatitis B is sometimes used to indicate the potential for the spread of HIV infection; injecting drug use and unprotected sexual activity are the most common routes of transmission for both.

* Factors such as:
1. The success of secondary prevention (e.g. partner notification).
2. The effectiveness of treatment.
3. Patterns of behaviour which may differ between different age cohorts but give the impression of showing change within a cohort over time.
4. The biological properties of the organism.
5. Other non-sexual routes of transmission.[24]

Sex education in schools

INTRODUCTION

Teenage pregnancy and abortion rates in the UK are high compared to other Western European countries, and this has raised concerns about the comprehensiveness and quality of sex education. In a recent survey carried out by the Family Planning Association 85 out of 110 pregnant 14–17-year-olds had not been to a family planning clinic or a GP for contraception. The most common reason, given by 66%, was that they thought it was illegal for under-16-year-olds. Knowledge of periods, pregnancy, HIV, condoms, other contraception and relationships was low.[1]

Although teenagers present to family doctors for the majority of health care, some teenagers find their GP unapproachable and are concerned about maintenance of confidentiality.[2,3]

Good practice in school health education to prevent AIDS and STDs has been encouraged by the World Health Organisation,[4] and sex education could play an important role in helping to reach the target set out in *The Health of the Nation*: to reduce by at least 50% the rate of conceptions amongst under-16s by the year 2000.[5]

A review of evaluations of the effectiveness of school-based sex education[6] concluded that programmes of sex education did not increase sexual activity. Rather, they delayed the onset of intercourse or had no effect; some can even increase the use of condoms and other contraceptives.

Findings from the National Survey of Sexual Attitudes and Lifestyles[7] confirm these effects. Men who reported learning about sex from school were less likely to have sex before the age of 16, and women were no more likely than those who reported learning about it from friends or the media. School sex education was linked to more responsible use of contraception.

Over six million young people between the ages of 5 and 19 attend the 23 000 schools in England[8] – thus schools provide direct access to a significant proportion of the population.

LEGISLATION

The place of sex education in the school curriculum has been the subject of discussion for some time. Changes introduced by section 241 of the Education Act 1993, came into force on 1 September 1994. Schools now have legal powers and duties summarised below:

in *maintained primary schools*, governing bodies have the responsibility of considering whether or at what stage to offer sex education. They must keep an up-to-date written statement of the policy they choose to adopt, which must be available to parents;

in *maintained secondary schools*, sex education (including education about HIV and AIDS and other sexually transmitted diseases) must be provided for all registered pupils. As in primary schools, the governing body must make a written statement of their policy on sex education available to all parents;

in *all maintained schools* any sex education must be provided in such a manner as to encourage young people to have regard to moral considerations and the value of family life. The parents of a pupil at any maintained school may, if they wish, withdraw that pupil from all or part of the sex education provided.[9]

Young people's entitlement to sexual health education can also be seen as a requirement of section 1(2) of the 1988 Reform Act which states that education 'should prepare pupils for the opportunities, responsibilities and experiences of adult life'.

The Department of the Environment clarified that section 28 of the Local Government Act (1988), which prohibits the promotion of homosexuality by local authorities, does *not* apply to schools; section 28 does not affect the activities of school governors, nor of teachers. It will not prevent the objective discussion of homosexuality in the classroom, nor the counselling of pupils concerned about their homosexuality (Department of the Environment Circular 12/88). This was reinforced in subsequent guidance to all schools in Circular 5/94 from the Department for Education.

Governing bodies of schools have no discretion as to whether the national curriculum should be taught – the law requires that it must be – but the inclusion of biological aspects of human behaviour in the Science Order does not mean that they must be taught within science lessons. Schools may, for example, prefer to include them within programmes of personal and social education.[10]*

* The main guidance document is Curriculum Guidance 5: Health Education.[10]

Attainment targets for all children (Key Stages 1, 2 and 3) and 14–16-year-olds (Key Stage 4) for science include topics relevant to sex education.[11]

SCHOOL SEX EDUCATION POLICIES

The existence of a sex education policy has been taken as an indicator of how seriously the subject of sex education is taken in schools. In an HEA survey of 1742 primary and secondary schools drawn from the Department of Education and Science register of schools in England in 1989, 61% of primary schools and 76% of secondary schools confirmed that they had a sex education policy. Schools with policies appeared to make greater use of teaching materials and training courses.[12]

Table 19 **Topics covered in sex education: England 1989**

	Primary %	Secondary %
Sex education	69	94
Relationships	81	94
HIV/AIDS	9	83
Child abuse	28	51
Drugs	41	92
Assertiveness	41	71
Self-esteem	68	86

Base: 1742 schools   Source: HEA [12]

Teachers were generally content with the quality and quantity of sex education given. Sixty-six per cent of teachers had received some training in aspects of health education although teachers in independent schools were significantly less likely to have done so. However, sex education was the most common area in health education in which teachers felt further training was needed.[12]

In a survey of 78% of all LEAs in England and Wales, 68% of teachers referred to uncertainty and embarrassment over the subject of sex education and 41% said teachers' time, curriculum time and resources were constraints to teaching the subject.[13] Several authors have concluded that more support and training for teachers is important.[14,15]

In a 1993 review of school policies in 798 schools, sex education was reported as being increasingly marginalised as schools put greater emphasis on national curriculum subjects. Two-thirds of schools that had appointed health co-ordinators were not able to give them enough time to carry out their work and suffered from a lack of resources for in-service training or new training materials. Schools also reported less support from health education co-ordinators, many of the posts having disappeared in recent years. The survey also suggested that the quality of sex education in schools was variable, with teachers preferring to give facts and information rather than teach the skills required for healthy relationships.[16]

ATTITUDES TO SEX EDUCATION
Young people

One in 10 students in a survey of 4436 16–19-year-olds reported never having been provided with information about sex. Eighty-four per cent reported learning about the physical development of bodies, pregnancy and contraception, but not about more controversial or sensitive subjects such as homosexuality or abortion.[17]

Only 55% reported having learnt about AIDS. Younger age groups, however, are more likely to report learning about AIDS, as the subject is taught more frequently every year.[17]

Sizeable proportions of the sample were dissatisfied with the amount of information they received and wanted to know more about abortion (38%), AIDS (44%) and other less discussed subjects such as homosexuality and lesbianism (45% and 46%).[17]

A more recent survey undertaken in 1995 by the HEA questioned 6406 schoolchildren aged 11, 13 and 15 years as part of an international survey of health within school-aged children.[18] Of seven health related topics, the one most commonly taught at school was sex education, the vast majority of 13- and 15-year-olds having received some sex education at school. However, the subject of HIV and AIDS was more likely to be taught to older pupils. At least 80% of 15-year-olds had attended classes covering sexual intercourse, safer sex, contraceptives, and HIV/AIDS. Young people generally found sexual topics much easier to discuss with friends of their own age than family members, teachers or health professionals. Teachers were especially seen as unapproachable amongst professionals by the young people in this survey.

The National AIDS Trust held a series of forums in 1991[19] in which 500 sixth-formers were asked to express their views on sex education. The following points summarise the views expressed:

● Too little sex education was provided too late

● Not enough time was given to discussion of issues about sex and sexuality

● Frustration was felt at the 'watering down' of information

● Videos should not be a substitute for discussion

● Less emphasis should be placed on facts and more on discussion and participation.

When 1025 15–16-years-olds were asked which sources had been most helpful in getting information about sex, school and friends were cited the most often and in almost equal proportions. Television was cited as the most helpful or next most helpful source of information about sexually transmitted diseases by 46% of the sample.[20]

Parents
The HEA's survey of 5007 adults found that 4 out of 5 think sex education in schools should include information on how to use a condom. There was widespread agreement in the survey that parents do not talk openly about sexual matters with their children, although those most likely to disagree were 16–19-year-olds and 35–54-year-olds.[21]

In a national survey of parental attitudes to sex education in schools 94% of 1462 respondents were supportive of school-based sex education. Parents saw the partnership between themselves and schools as the essential pre-condition for effectively meeting the needs of their children.[22]

Appendices

APPENDIX 1: SOCIAL GRADING SYSTEMS

Many scales have been devised to give a precise definition of socioeconomic grouping for research. Classification is by current or former occupation of head of household in the two most widely used systems – the Registrar-General's social class system, used in the Census and the National Readership Survey system used by most UK market research.

NRS System	Registrar-General (OPCS)	Description	Examples
A	I	Professional/Upper middle class	professor, doctor bank manager
B	II	Intermediate/Middle class	journalist, nurse, teacher
C1	IIIN	Skilled non-manual/Lower middle class	clerical worker, shop assistant
C2	IIIM	Skilled manual/Skilled working class	bus driver, miner, carpenter
D	IV V	Partly skilled/Unskilled working class	agricultural worker, hospital porter, labourer, cleaner, dock worker
E		Those at lowest levels of subsistence	old-age pensioner, widows, and those totally dependent on social security through long-term unemployment and sickness

As the table shows, the two systems are roughly comparable. However, the Registrar-General's system classifies the retired and unemployed by their last significant period of employment, but the ABC system merges groups IV and V into D and creates an additional category E for those dependent on social security and state pensions. The scales are unsatisfactory for several reasons: married women are classified by their husband's occupation rather than their own; there can be quite marked lifestyle differences within occupational groups; and grading systems can vary slightly between different market research agencies.

APPENDIX 2: DISCOVERY AND BIOLOGY OF HIV AND AIDS

HIV

The virus now known as HIV-1 was first isolated in 1983 by a team of researchers working in Paris.[1] Initially they called the virus lymphadenopathy-associated virus (LAV) because it was isolated from tissue from a gay man with persistently swollen lymph glands. Researchers in the United States isolated the same virus but termed it human T-cell lymphotropic virus Type III (HTLV III).[2–5] Subsequently, the virus was renamed human immunodeficiency virus (HIV).

Viruses can only reproduce themselves inside living cells. They invade host cells, and, using their own DNA or RNA,* instruct the cell to make new copies of the virus. HIV is a retrovirus,[1] that is a virus that holds its genetic information in the form of RNA rather than DNA. HIV attacks in particular CD4 lymphocytes. Lymphocytes are white blood cells vital to the body's immune reactions; T lymphocytes with CD4 receptor molecules are known as CD4 lymphocytes (also CD4 cells or helper T cells).

HIV infection leads to a progressive depletion of the number of CD4 lymphocytes. Although the precise mechanism of cell depletion is still unclear, progress has been made in understanding viral-host dynamics. HIV can also infect some other cells of the immune system and some brain tissue cells. In recent years, a number of individuals with what appears to be natural immunity have been identified.[6]

HIV-1 was the first strain of the virus to be isolated and characterised. Another strain, HIV-2, was discovered in 1986 and is endemic in West Africa, with limited distribution elsewhere. HIV-2 is less efficiently transmitted than HIV-1, but also causes AIDS. HIV is genetically variable, and both strains contain a variety of subtypes, different ones of which predominate in different parts of the world.[7] Although they are all spread by the same routes, research is underway into the relative efficiency of different modes of transmission.[8]

There is still no vaccine against HIV.

DNA – (deoxyribonucleic acid C) and RNA (ribonucleic acid C) constitute the genetic material of all living things. DNA is capable of replication, thus enabling all the hereditary information contained in the genetic code to be passed on.

AIDS

AIDS (acquired immune deficiency syndrome) was first recognised as a new and distinct clinical entity in 1981.[9–11] The first cases were recognised because of an unusual clustering of diseases such as Kaposi's sarcoma (KS) and *Pneumocystis carinii* pneumonia (PCP) in young homosexual men. Originally, AIDS was defined as a syndrome diagnosed by the presence of one or more very specific diseases that rarely affect persons with a normal immune response.

The case definition used for AIDS has changed over time. The European AIDS case definition for surveillance[12] follows the 1993 Centers for Disease Control and Prevention (CDC) definition. The main difference is that it does not include CD4 count as a defining condition.

There is an asymptomatic period of variable length (median 10 to 11 years in adults) before people with HIV develop severe immune deficiency.[13] It is not clear why this period varies for different individuals. Few data are available beyond 12 years but it is expected that the vast majority of HIV-1 infected persons will develop AIDS eventually. Research into people with exceptionally lengthy asymptomatic stages ('long-term non-progressors') may yield some answers.[14]

Virtually all persons diagnosed as having AIDS die within a few years. Survival after diagnosis has been increasing in industrialised countries from an average of less than 1 year to about 1–2 years at present. A study of 3984 AIDS patients in the UK showed that survival patterns have been changing and generally improving (one-third of the patients had been surviving for 2 years or more) which may be due to more prompt diagnosis and improved treatment.[15] However survival time with AIDS in developing countries remains short – an estimated 6 months or less; reasons for this have not been fully established.

APPENDIX 3: COLLECTION OF DATA ON HIV AND AIDS

AIDS and HIV surveillance

How data are compiled in England and Wales

The AIDS Control Act (1987) requires health authorities and health boards to report each year the number of people with AIDS known to them.

Data on HIV infection and AIDS are compiled by the Public Health Laboratory Service's (PHLS) AIDS Centre at the Communicable Diseases Surveillance Centre (CDSC), and the Scottish Centre for Infection and Environmental Health (SCIEH).[1] In addition data on HIV positive children are collated at the Institute of Child Health, London (ICH-L) in collaboration with CDSC and SCIEH.

Surveillance includes the following:

(a) Voluntary confidential reporting of AIDS cases and deaths in HIV-infected persons by clinicians.

(b) Voluntary confidential reporting of newly-identified HIV infections by microbiologists.

   For AIDS cases, deaths in HIV-infected persons and HIV infection reports, the information held confidentially by the PHLS will included a soundex unique identifier code, the sex and age of the person, an assessment of how they acquired HIV and, if available, their ethnic group.

(c) The PHLS Collaborative Laboratory Study recording all HIV tests (both positive and negative) in 17 sentinel laboratories in England and Wales (with a parallel study in Scotland). This monitors variations in numbers, exposure categories, and trends in HIV prevalence in persons tested for HIV infection.

(d) Unlinked anonymous HIV surveillance (see below).

(e) Voluntary confidential reporting of HIV infection in pregnancy by obstetricians and HIV in children by paediatricians via the RCOG and BPASU respectively.

In addition to this, PHLS takes other data into account in describing the epidemiology of HIV, e.g. blood donor screening, which indicates the extent of HIV infection in groups not at major risk of infection.

Data on sexually transmitted diseases (STDs) and sexual behaviour are also important in order to understand the spread of HIV infection in the UK (see related chapters). CDSC also make use of hepatitis B and tuberculosis surveillance reports, opportunistic infection reports and mortality trends in selected age groups. Data from other countries provide an international perspective.[2]

Presentation

A range of summary data are published each month by the PHLS in the *Communicable Disease Report*.

These include cumulative totals for AIDS and HIV infection reports (i.e. the number of reports since recording began, which is 1982 for AIDS and 1984 for HIV) and the number of reports of HIV and AIDS cases reported in the last quarter and the last 12 months.

An annual report is published by the Department of Health, CDSC and ICH-L for the unlinked anonymous programme and projections reports are produced at roughly 3-year intervals.

Interpreting the statistics

Care should be taken with the interpretation of AIDS and HIV statistics. Unlike morbidity and mortality data for other diseases, cumulative totals are given which include all reports since recording began. The HIV totals will include some of those people who have progressed to AIDS (and possibly died) and the AIDS totals include those who have died. PHLS records separately the number who have died, but does not subtract this from their cumulative total of AIDS cases.

The most important use of AIDS statistics is to assist those planning care for people with AIDS. A limitation of AIDS statistics is that there is a median time period of 10 years between infection with HIV and development of AIDS. The PHLS estimate that under-reporting of AIDS cases is around 13%. There will also be under-reporting of deaths because in some circumstances AIDS-related death may not be mentioned on a death certificate because of social stigma.

HIV infection reports can be used for planning purposes but it should be remembered that they reflect test uptake and test date rather than actual numbers of HIV infections. The cumulative number of HIV infection reports is not the total number of HIV-infected persons. Reasons for this include the fact that there will be people who are unaware that they are infected, and who have not been tested because they do not recognise themselves to be at risk; there are people who may recognise that they are at risk but decide not to be tested; there will be a few people who may have

been tested during the 'window' (3 months) period before their immune system formed antibodies, and therefore were found to be antibody negative (and did not return for a second test).

Unlinked anonymous surveillance

Since 1990, a programme of unlinked anonymous HIV prevalence monitoring has been under way in the UK. The primary purpose of these surveys is to provide trend data on those whose behaviour makes them vulnerable to HIV infection and those at more general risk. These serosurveys minimise the effects of participation bias (inherent in the voluntary testing system) and therefore allow the prevalence of infection to be estimated more accurately. The primary purpose of unlinked anonymous surveillance is to monitor trends in prevalence of HIV infection among adults whose behaviour makes them vulnerable (persons who inject drugs and/or have had higher levels of partner change). All specimens are irreversibly unlinked from any identification before testing so that individual tests cannot be traced back to the source patient.

APPENDIX 4: DEFINITIONS AND SEQUELAE OF STDs

Herpes
Herpes simplex 2 is the virus causing genital herpes. (However, herpes simplex 1, which causes cold sores, also causes some infection.)

Most frequent among 20–24-year-olds, genital herpes is thought to increase the risk of HIV transmission because of ulceration.

Symptoms include small painful blisters appearing on or around the genital area; tingling or itching in the genital area; general flu-like symptoms such as headache, backache or a temperature and pain or burning sensation when passing urine.

Treatment: No cure is available at present although an anti-viral drug (acyclovir) can minimise the severity and length of first attacks. It has little effect on recurrences, but these are normally infrequent and short-lived. Genital herpes may lead to cell changes in the cervix; infected women should have annual smears, as advised by their doctor or clinic.

Transmission: Close body contact, sexual intercourse and oral sex (via cold sores).
Sequelae: Recurrences can spread to other parts of the body and cause complications in the central nervous system, but these are rare.

Genital warts
Caused by the human papilloma virus, genital warts have been of concern primarily because of the virus's association with pre-cancerous cell changes in the cervix. Genital warts are one of the most common STDs and are more common amongst 16–25-year-olds.

Warts do not necessarily appear immediately after infection and cannot always be seen easily, especially if they occur inside the vagina, particularly the cervix, or anus.

Treatment: Local application of ointments or paints (e.g. podophyllin), freezing, or surgical removal under local anaesthetic. Women who have had warts or whose partners have had warts should have annual smear tests.

Transmission: Close body contact, sexual intercourse and oral sex.
Sequelae: Possibly cervical cancer. In rare cases, infants may contract the virus at birth.

Syphilis
Syphilis is caused by the *Treponema pallidum* bacterium. As the bacteria cannot survive in the open air it is nearly always transmitted sexually. Historically known as 'the pox', syphilis is not very common nowadays. Symptoms are a painless sore usually on or near the vagina or penis but sometimes in the mouth or anus, followed by a rash on the body and flu-like symptoms.

Treatment: Antibiotics can cure syphilis completely.
Transmission: Close body contact, sexual intercourse and oral sex.
Sequelae: Eventually attacks the nervous system and can cause blindness (though this is rare), heart problems and dementia. Syphilis can be contracted *in utero* in the later stages of pregnancy, causing still births, severe cardiovascular and neurological disease (notably deafness) and infant death.

Gonorrhoea
Caused by the gonococcus bacterium, *Neisseria gonorrhoeae*, gonorrhoea is more common amongst younger adults. (Gonorrhoea has sometimes been known as 'the clap'.) Symptoms are different for men and women. Most women with gonorrhoea do not have any symptoms. The main symptom for men is a urethral discharge, as well as a burning pain on passing urine, occasionally an irritation or discharge from the anus. Gonorrhoea passed on during oral sex may cause a sore throat. Anal gonorrhoea is more common in homosexual men.

Treatment: Antibiotics.
Transmission: Intimate body contact, sexual intercourse and oral sex.
Sequelae: Can cause pelvic inflammatory disease. Pregnant mothers can infect children, causing gonococcal conjunctivitis. Amongst men, it can inflame the testicles, causing abscesses that can result in the loss of a testicle.

Non-specific genital infection (NSGI)
This is a large group of different infections which are among the most common of all STDs. They include vaginitis (inflammation of the vagina), urethritis (inflammation of the urethra), cystitis (inflammation of the bladder) and proctitis (inflammation of the rectum).

The term NSGI is often used when the infection is not known and it may include chlamydia where tests are not done for this (often in men). NSGI occurs when bacteria normally present in small numbers in the genitals multiply.

Symptoms include discharge from the vagina, urethra, penis or anus; inflammation around the genital area, desire to pass urine more frequently, pain or burning sensation on passing urine.

Many women, however, do not notice any symptoms.

Treatment: Antibiotics.
Transmission: Can be sexually transmitted.
Sequelae: Can cause pelvic inflammatory disease (PID) and possibly infertility.

Chlamydia

This is caused by *Chlamydia trachomatis* and is a very common bacterial STD in industrialised countries. There are often no visible signs of chlamydia but women may have a vaginal discharge or pain when passing urine if the urethra is inflamed. Men may have symptoms of non-specific urethritis (NSU).

Treatment: Antibiotics.
Transmission: Sexual intercourse.
Sequelae: Chlamydia is one of the infections which, if left untreated, can cause pelvic inflammatory disease (PID), which can cause infertility. In men urethritis caused by chlamydia (non-specific urethritis – NSU) is a warning signal for a more serious infection of a female partner. It is thought that about one-third of male infertility is probably caused by chlamydia.

Trichomoniasis

Caused by tiny parasites (trichonomads), trichomoniasis infects the vagina and the urethra. Men usually have no symptoms; women have a discharge, itching and irritation.

Although it is not a serious condition, trichomoniasis is often diagnosed with gonorrhoea and can be a warning signal for a more serious gonococcal infection.

Treatment: Antibiotics.
Transmission: Close body contact and sexual intercourse.
Sequelae: None.

Candidiasis *(thrush)*

Caused by *Candida albicans*, a yeast which is often present in the vagina but which can multiply beyond normal levels. Symptoms in women include a thick, white discharge from the vagina, possible swelling of the vulva, soreness and pain on passing urine and itching around the genital or anal area. Men may experience inflammation of the penis.

Treatment: Pessaries and cream for women (also natural remedies such as live yoghurt), cream for men.
Transmission: Is not necessarily sexual and can be triggered by antibiotics, some forms of contraceptive and sexual activity, although infection can occur during sex.
Sequelae: None.

Pubic lice *(Pediculosis pubis)*

These are tiny crab-like creatures which live in pubic hair and causing itching.

Treatment: Liquid solutions such as Prioderm or Quelleda.
Transmission: Close body contact not necessarily sexual, or via towels and bedclothes, etc.
Sequelae: None; but the lice can spread to other parts of the body.

Scabies

Caused by *Sarcoptes scabiei*.

Treatment: Benzyl benzoate emulsion.
Transmission: Close body contact, towels, bedclothes, etc.
Sequelae: No serious health implication but the infection will spread. Persistent widespread itching.

Hepatitis B

Hepatitis means 'inflammation of the liver'. There are a number of different types of hepatitis, including A, B, and C. Type B is caused by the hepatitis B virus (HBV).

The first stage of symptoms (which may appear between one and six months after contact with the infection) are flu-like, a severe feeling of tiredness and loss of appetite and pain in the joints, followed by jaundice.

Treatment: No specific treatment available, very severe cases may be hospitalised but most patients recover completely after a period of bed rest.
Prevention: There is a vaccine against hepatitis B, available at GUM clinics.
Transmission: Can be spread through sexual contact and contact with body fluids such as blood, saliva and urine. (HBV is much more infectious than HIV.)
Sequelae: May cause long-term liver damage.

APPENDIX 5: SURVEYS QUOTED

Title	Date	Sample size	Area covered
Project Sigma (Socio-Sexual Investigations of Gay Men and AIDS) Longitudinal study of a cohort of homosexually active men aged 15–81 recruited in 1987–88 and re-interviewed, on average every 10 months.	1987–93	930	England and Wales
British Social Attitudes Survey (SCPR) Interviews with adults aged 18 or over.	1983–89	1610–1274	Britain
General Household Survey (OPCS) Interviews with women aged 16–49.	1994	5571	Britain
The Socio-sexual Lifestyles of Young People Living in the South West of England Interviews with 16–24-year-olds.	1989–90	3777	South-west of England
The National Survey of Sexual Attitudes and Lifestyles Interviews with adults aged 16–59.	1990–91	18 876	Britain
AIDS Research in Gay Bars (Carried out by BMRB on behalf of the HEA) Interviews with male gay bar attenders.	1986–96	c.300 per year 333 in 1996	England and Scotland
AIDS Strategic Monitor (Carried out by BMRB on behalf of the HEA) Interviews with adults aged 13 and over.	1991	1686	UK
Advertising Monitor (Carried out by BMRB on behalf of the HEA) Interviews with adults aged 16–54.	1993	600–1500	Britain (boosts, UK)
Today's Young Adults (Carried out by MORI on behalf of the HEA) Interviews with 16-19-year-olds.	1990	4436	England
Health and Lifestyles Survey (Carried out by MORI on behalf of the HEA) Self-completed questionnaires.	1992	4000	UK
Black and Ethnic Minority Communities Health and Lifestyle Survey (Carried out by MORI on behalf of the HEA) Interviews with Indians, Pakistanis and Bangladeshis.	1992	Asians 2609 General population 5007	England
Consumer Choices in Family Planning (University of Exeter, Institute of Population Studies) Interviews with 18–44-year-olds.	1991	2147	England
Health Education Monitoring Survey (carried out by ONS on behalf of the HEA) Interviews with 16–74-year-olds.	1995	4672	England

Britain comprises England, Scotland and Wales. UK comprises Britain and Northern Ireland.

References

Introduction

1. World Health Organization, 1974. Quoted in *AIDS Action*, 1991, issue 13, p1.

2. Department of Health. *Health of the Nation: a Strategy for Health in England*, Cm 1986. HMSO, 1992.

Sexual behaviour

1. Johnson, A. and Wadsworth, J. *et al.* Sexual lifestyles and HIV risk. *Nature*, **360**, 1992, pp 410–11.

2. Wellings, K. *et al. Sexual behaviour in Britain: the national survey of sexual attitudes and lifestyles.* Penguin Books, 1994.

3. Bridgwood, A. *et al. Health in England, 1995: What people know, what people think, what people do.* London: ONS, 1996.

4. Business Monitor. *Overseas travel and tourism 1988.* Central Statistical Office: 1989; MA6:1–720.

5. PHLS AIDS Centre, CDSC and Scottish Centre for Infection and Environmental Health. AIDS/HIV quarterly surveillance tables, unpublished, No. 31, March 1996.

6. Gostin, L. O. *et al.* Screening international travellers for the human immunodeficiency virus. *New England Journal of Medicine*, **322**, 1990, pp 1743–6.

7. Gillies, P. *et al.* HIV-related risk behaviour in UK holiday makers. *AIDS*, **3**, 1992, pp 339–42.

8. Noone, A. Gill, O. N. *et al.* Travel, heterosexual intercourse and HIV-1 infection. *Communicable Disease Review*, **1** (4), 1991, R39–R43.

9. Steffen, R. *et al.* Casual sexual contacts of Swiss tourists in tropical Africa, the Far East and Latin America. Fifth International Conference on AIDS, Montreal, 1989. Abstract M.D.P. p 25.

10. Behrens, R. H. and Porter, J. D. H. HIV infection and foreign travel. *British Medical Journal*, **301**, 1990, p 1217.

11. Hawkes, S. J. *et al.* A study of the prevalence of HIV infection and associated risk factors in international travellers. Poster presentation at the VIII International Conference on AIDS/III STD World Review, Amsterdam 19–24 July 1992.

12. HEA/NOP. *Young travellers and HIV prevention.* London, 1995.

13. Hawkes, S. *et al.* Risk behaviour and HIV prevalence in international travellers, *AIDS*, **8**, 1994, pp 247–52.

14. Rhodes, T. and Stimson, G. V. What is the relationship between drug taking and sexual risk? Social relations and social research. *Sociology of Health and Illness*, 1994, **16** (2), pp 209-28.

15. Weatherburn, P. *et al.* No connection between alcohol use and safe sex among gay and bisexual men. *AIDS*, **7**, 1993, pp 115–19.

16. Bagnall, G. and Plant, M. A. HIV/AIDS risks, alcohol and illicit drug use among young adults in areas of high and low rates of HIV infection. *AIDS Care*, **3** (4), 1991, pp 355–61.

17. Robertson, J. A. and Plant, M. A. Alcohol, sex and risks of HIV infection. *Drugs and Alcohol Dependence*, **22**, 1988, pp 75–8.

18. Plant, M. A. and Plant, M. L. *Risk-takers: alcohol, drugs, sex and youth.* London: Routledge, 1992.

19. Bureau of Hygiene and Tropical Diseases. *AIDS Newsletter*, **8** (10), 1993, p 20. Conference Report on IX International Conference on AIDS/HIV/STD World Congress, Berlin, Germany, 6–11 June 1993.

20. Donoghoe, M *et al.* Sexual behaviour of injecting drug users and associated risks of HIV infection for non-injecting sexual partners. *AIDS Care,* **1** (1), 1989, pp 51–8.

21. Klee, H. *et al.* AIDS-related risk behaviour, poly-drug use and temazepam. *British Journal of Addiction*, **85**, 1990, pp 1125–32.

22. Mulleady, G. and Sherr, L. Lifestyle factors for drug users in relation to risks for HIV. *AIDS Care,* **1** (1) 1989, pp 45–50.

23. Gossop, M. *et al.* Severity of heroin dependence and HIV risk. 1 Sexual behaviour. *AIDS Care,* **5** (2), 1993, pp 149–57.

24. Strang, J. *et al.* Heterosexual vaginal and anal intercourse amongst London heroine and cocaine users. *International Journal of STD and AIDS*, **5**, 1994, pp 133–6.

25. Hunter, G. *et al.* Changes in the injecting risk behaviour of injecting drug users in London, 1990-93. *AIDS*, **9**, 1995, pp 493–501.

26. Bureau of Hygiene and Tropical Diseases. *AIDS Newsletter*, **7** (12), 1992, p 37.

27. Klee, H. Heroin and amphetamine users compared. *Addiction*, **88** (8), 1993, pp 1055–62.

28. Plant, M. The sex industry, alcohol and illicit drugs: implications for the spread of HIV infection. *British Journal of Addiction*, **84**, 1989, pp 53–9.

29. Ward, H. *et al.* Prostitution and risk of HIV, in female prostitutes in London. *British Medical Journal*, **307**, 1993, pp 356–8.

30. Gossop, M. *et al.* Female prostitutes in South London: use of heroin, cocaine and alcohol and their relationship to health risk behaviours. *AIDS Care,* **7** (3), 1995, pp 253–60.

31. McKeganey, N. Selling sex: female prostitution and HIV risk behaviour in Glasgow. *AIDS Care,* **4** (4), 1992, pp 395–407.

32. McKeganey, N. *et al.* A comparison of HIV related risk behaviour and risk reduction between female street prostitutes and male rent boys in Glasgow. *Sociology of Health and Illness,* **12**, 1990, pp 274–92.

33. Gossop, M. *et al.* Sexual behaviour and its relationship to drug taking among prostitutes in south London. *Addiction,* **89**, 1994, pp 961-70.

34. PHLS CDSC. AIDS and HIV infection in the United Kingdom: monthly report. *Communicable Disease Report,* **6** (16), 1996.

35. Chu, S. Y. *et al.* Female-to-female sexual contact and HIV transmission. *Journal of the American Medical Association,* **272** (6), 1994, p 433.

36. Health Education Authority. *Monitoring AIDS: ten years of gay bar surveys 1986–1996.* Report on a series of quantitative surveys carried out by BMRB on behalf of the HEA. In press, 1997.

37. Davis, T.M. *et al. Sex, gay men and AIDS.* London: Falmer, 1993.

38. Hickson, F. (Project SIGMA) *Sexual exclusivity, non exclusivity and HIV.* Project SIGMA Working Paper No. 31. (1992), London: Project SIGMA.

39. Stall, R. *et al.* Alcohol and drug use during sexual activity and compliance with safe sex guidelines for AIDS: the AIDS Behavioural Research Project. *Health Education,* **13** (4), 1986, pp 359–72.

40. Davies, P. and Feldman, R. *Male sex workers in South Wales.* Project SIGMA Working Paper No. 15. (1993), London: Project SIGMA.

41. Sigma Research and the Health Education Authority. *Behaviourally bisexual men in the UK: identifying needs for HIV prevention.* London: HEA, 1996.

42. Hunt, A. J. *et al.* Changes in sexual behaviour in a large cohort of homosexual men in England and Wales, 1988–89, *British Medical Journal,* **302**, 1991, pp 505–6.

43. Health Education Authority. *AIDS Strategic Monitor* (January 1990 – February 1991) survey carried out by BMRB on behalf of the HEA. London: HEA, 1994.

44. Health Education Authority. *Health and lifestyle survey: a survey of the UK population,* Part 1. Carried out by MORI on behalf of the HEA. London: HEA, 1995.

45. Health Education Authority. *Today's young adults: 16–19-year-olds look at diet, alcohol, smoking, drugs and sexual behaviour.* London: HEA, 1992.

46. Ford, N. *The socio-sexual lifestyles of young people in the South West of England.* South Western Regional Health Authority and University of Exeter, 1991.

47. Bury, J. K. *Teenage pregnancy in Britain.* London: Birth Control Trust, 1989.

48. Health Education Authority. *Talking about it: young people, sexual behaviour and HIV.* London: HEA, 1993.

49. Macintyre, S. and West, P. What does the phrase 'safer sex' mean to you? - understanding among Glaswegian 18-year-olds in 1990. *AIDS,* **7**, 1992, pp 121–5.

50. Department of Health. Statistical Bulletin 1996/4. *Sexually transmitted diseases, England, 1995: new cases seen at NHS genito-urinary medicine clinics.*

51. Cancer Research Campaign. *Cancer of the cervix uteri.* Factsheet 12.3. Cancer Research Campaign, 1990.

Conceptions

1. Office for National Statistics. *Conceptions in England and Wales, 1994.* Series FM1 96/2. ONS, 1996.

2. Department of Health. *The health of the nation: a strategy for health in England.* Cm 1986. HMSO, 1992.

3. Metson, D. Lessons from an audit of unplanned pregnancies. *British Medical Journal,* **297**, 1988, pp 904–6.

4. Fleissig, A. Family planning services – use and preferences of recent mothers. *British Journal of Family Planning,* **17**, 1992, pp 110–14.

5. Cartwright, A. Unintended pregnancy that leads to babies. *Social Science and Medicine,* **27**, 1988, pp 249–54.

6. Royal College of Obstetricians and Gynaecologists. *Report of the RCOG Working Party on Unplanned Pregnancy.* London: RCOG, 1991.

7. Simms, M. and Smith, C. *Teenage mothers and their partners: a survey in England and Wales.* HMSO, 1986.

8. Family Planning Association. *Children who have children.* FPA, 1993.

9. Russell, J. *Early teenage pregnancy.* Churchill Livingstone, 1982.

10. Fraser A. M. *et al.* Association of young maternal age with adverse reproductive outcomes, *New England Journal of Medicine,* **332**, 1995, pp 1113–17.

11. Murphy J. F. *et al.* Cardiff Birth Survey. *Journal of Epidemiology and Community Health,* **36**, 1982, pp 17–21.

12. Makinson, C. The health consequences of teenage fertility. *Family Planning Perspectives,* **17** (3), 1985, pp 132–9.

13. Geronimus, A. T. and Korenman, S. Maternal youth or family background? On the health disadvantages of infants with teenage mothers. *American Journal of Epidemiology,* **137**, 1993, pp 213–25.

14. Babb, P. Teenage conceptions and fertility in England and Wales, 1971–1991. *Population Trends,* **74**, 1993, pp 12–17.

15. Munday D. *et al.* Twenty one years of legal abortion. *British Medical Journal,* **298**, 1989, pp 1231–4.

16. Office of Population Censuses and Surveys. *Birth Statistics 1992: England and Wales.* Series FM1, No. 21. London: HMSO, 1994.

17. Office for National Statistics. *Birth Statistics 1994: England and Wales.* Series FM1, No. 23. London: HMSO, 1996.

18. Council of Europe. Recent demographic developments in Europe. 1994.

19. Jones, E. F. *et al.* Teenage pregnancy in developed countries: determinants and policy implications. *Family Planning Perspectives,* **17**, 1985, pp 53–63.

20. Jones, E. F. *et al. Teenage pregnancy in developed countries: determinants and policy implications.* A study funded by the Alan Guttmacher Institute. New Haven: Yale University Press, 1986.

21. Wilson, S. *et al.* Teenage conceptions and contraception in English regions. *Journal of Public Health Medicine,* **14**, 1992, pp 17–25.

22. Kiernan, K. Teenage motherhood – associated factors and consequences – the experiences of a British cohort. *Journal of Biosocial Science,* **12**, 1980, pp 393–405.

23. Garlick, R. *et al.* The UPA score and teenage pregnancy. *Public Health,* **107**, 1993, pp 135–9.

24. McGuire, A. and Hughes, D. *The economics of family planning services: a report prepared by the Contraceptive Alliance.* London: Family Planning Association, 1995.

25. Office for National Statistics. Monitor. *Live births in England and Wales.* Series FM1 96/1. ONS, 1996.

26. Office for National Statistics. Monitor. *Legal abortions in England and Wales, 1995.* Series AB 96/5, ONS, 1996.

Contraception

1. Bone, M. *Family planning services in England and Wales.* HMSO, 1973.

2. Bone, M. *The family planning services: changes and effects.* HMSO, 1978.

3. Dunnell, K. *Family formation 1976.* HMSO, 1979.

4. Office of Population Censuses and Surveys. *General Household Survey 1983.* HMSO, 1985.

5. Office of Population Censuses and Surveys. *General Household Survey 1993.* HMSO, 1995.

6. Schering Health Care. Press release. 'What women really think about sex and contraception'. Survey carried out by National Opinion Polls on behalf of Schering Health Care. Schering, 1993.

7. Wellings, K. *et al. Sexual health in Britain: the national survey of sexual attitudes and lifestyles.* Penguin Books, 1994.

8. Blacksell, S. *et al. Consumer choices in family planning.* University of Exeter, 1992.

9. McAvoy, B. R. Asian women: (i) Contraceptive knowledge, attitudes and usage. *Health Trends,* **20**, 1988, pp 11–17.

10. Woollett, A. The attitudes to contraception among Asian women in east London. *British Journal of Family Planning,* **17**, 1991, pp 72–7.

11. Beard, P. Contraception in ethnic minority groups in Bedford. *Health Visitor,* **55**, 1982, pp 417–22.

12. Health Education Authority. *Health and lifestyle survey (Black and Minority Ethnic Communities 1992).* London: HEA, 1994. Data quoted are provisional.

13. Royal College of General Practitioners' Oral Contraceptive Study. Mortality among oral-contraceptive users. *Lancet,* ii (8041), 1977, pp 727–33.

14. Vessey, M. P. *et al.* Mortality among women participating in the Oxford/FPA Contraceptive Study. *Lancet,* ii (8041), 1977, pp 731–3.

15. Pike, M. C. *et al.* Breast cancer in young women and use of oral contraceptives: possible modifying effect of formulation and age at use. *Lancet,* ii (8356), 1983, pp 926–30.

16. Vessey, M. P. *et al.* Neoplasia of the cervix uteri: a possible adverse effect of the pill. *Lancet,* ii (8356), 1983, pp 930–4.

17. Bromham, D. R. Pill prevents cancer! *British Journal of Family Planning,* **15**, 1989, p 35.

18. Kakouris, H. Pill failure in non-use of secondary precautions. *The British Journal of Family Planning,* **18**, 1992, pp 41–4.

19. Duncan, G. *et al.* Termination of pregnancy: lessons for prevention. *British Journal of Family Planning*, **15**, 1990, pp 112–17.

20. Brook, S. J. and Smith, C. Do combined oral contraceptive users know how to take their pill correctly? *British Journal of Family Planning*, **17**, 1991, pp 18–20.

21. Ford, N. *The socio-sexual lifestyles of young people in the South West of England.* South Western Regional Health Authority & University of Exeter, 1991.

22. Committee on Safety of Medicines. Combined oral contraceptives and thromboembolism. Letter to doctors and pharmacists, 18 October 1995.

23. Armstrong, J. L. *et al.* Effect on women attending a family planning clinic. *British Medical Journal*, **311**, 1995, p 1111 (letter).

24. Abortions rise after pill scare. *Abortion Review*, **59**, 1996, p 6.

25. Wellings, K. Trends in contraceptive method usage since 1970. *British Journal of Family Planning*, **12**, 1986, pp 15–22.

26. Family Planning Association. *Methods of contraception: past, present and future.* Factsheet 3A. FPA, 1992.

27. UK Family Planning Research Network. Condom use and patterns of sexual behaviour among sexually experienced women attending family planning clinics in England, Scotland and Wales. *British Journal of Family Planning*, **15** (3), 1989, pp 75–80.

28. Bridgwood, A. *et al. Health in England 1995: What people know, what people think, what people do.* Health Education Authority. London: ONS, 1996.

29. Bounds, W. *et al.* Female condom (Femidom™). A clinical study of its use – effectiveness and patient acceptability. *British Journal of Family Planning*, **18**, 1992, pp 36–41.

30. Ford, N. and Mathie, E. The acceptability and experience of the female condom: Femidom among family planning users. *British Journal of Family Planning*, **19**, 1993, pp 187–92.

31. Master, L. *et al.* How do attenders of a genitourinary medicine clinic feel about the female condom? *British Journal of Family Planning*, **21**, 1996, pp 135–38.

32. Health Education Authority. *Today's young adults: 16–19-year-olds look at diet, alcohol, smoking, drugs and sexual behaviour.* London: HEA, 1992.

33. Bury, J. K. *Teenage pregnancy in Britain.* London: Birth Control Trust, 1989.

34. British Medical Association, GMSC, Health Education Authority, Brook Advisory Centres, Family Planning Association and Royal College of General Practitioners. *Confidentiality & people under 16: guidance issued jointly by BMA, GMSC, HEA, Brook Advisory Centres, FPA and RCGP.* BMA, 1993.

35. Family Planning Association. *Your guide to contraception.* FPA, 1993.

36. World Health Organisation. *Oral contraceptives: technical and safety aspects.* Geneva: WHO, 1982.

37. Back, D. J. *et al.* Clinical pharmacology of O.C. steroid: drug interactions. *Journal of Obstetrics and Gynaecology*, **1**, 1980, pp 126–38.

38. Sapire, K. E. *Contraception and sexuality in health and disease.* UK edition revised and adapted by T. Belfield, and J. Guillebaud. London: McGraw-Hill, 1990.

39. Hatcher, R. Contraceptive failure rates. In: R. A. Hatcher (ed.) *Contraceptive technology*, 16th edn. New York: Irvington, 1994, pp 637–87.

40. Farr, G. *et al.* Contraceptive efficacy and acceptability of the female condom. *American Journal of Public Health,* **84**, 1994, pp 1960–64.

41. Which? Condoms on test. *Which? Way to Health*, August 1993, pp 119–23. (Consumers' Association)

42. Cates, W. and Stone, K. M. Family planning, sexually transmitted diseases and contraceptive choice: a literature update – parts I & II. *Family Planning Perspectives*, **24**, 1992, pp 75–84 and pp 123–8.

43. Minuk, G. Y. *et al.* Condoms and prevention of AIDS. *Journal of the American Medical Association*, **256**, 1986, p 1443.

44. Weller, S. C. A meta-analysis of condom effectiveness in reducing sexually transmitted HIV. *Social Science and Medicine*, 36 (12), 1993, pp 1635–14.

45. Syrjanen, K. *et al.* Sexual behaviour of women with human papillomavirus (HPV) lesions of the uterine cervix. *British Journal of Venereal Diseases*, **60**, 1984, p 243.

46. Leeper, M. A. *et al.* Preliminary evaluation of Reality, a condom for women to wear. *Advances in Contraception*, **55**, 1989, pp 229–35.

47. Soper, *et al.* Prevention of vagina trichomonas by compliant use of the female condom. *Sexually Transmitted Diseases*, **20**, 1993, pp 137–9.

48. Hooton, T. M. *et al.* Escherichia coli bacteriuria and contraceptive methods, *Journal of the American Medical Association*, **265**, 1991, pp 64–9.

49. Louv, W. C. *et al.* A clinical trial of nonoxynol-9 as a prophylaxis for cervical neisseria gonorrhoea and chlamydia trachomatis infections. *Journal of Infectious Diseases*, **158**, 1988, pp 518–23.

50. Kelaghan, J. *et al.* Barrier-method contraceptives and pelvic inflammatory disease. *Journal of the American Medical Association*, **248**, 1982, p 184.

51. Cavalieri d'Oro, L. *et al.* Barrier methods of contraception, spermicides, and sexually transmitted diseases: a review. *Genitourinary Medicine,* **70**, 1994, pp 410–17.

52. Alcorn, K. (ed.) *AIDS reference manual*. London: NAM Publications, 1996.

53. Austin, H. *et al.* A case-control study of spermicides and gonorrhoea. *Journal of the American Medical Association*, **251**, 1984, pp 2822–4.

54. Rosenberg, M. J. *et al.* Barrier contraceptives and sexually transmitted diseases in women: a comparison of female-dependent methods and condoms. *American Journal of Public Health*, **82** (5), 1992, pp 669–74.

55. Kjaer, S. K. *et al.* Risk factors for cervical human papillomavirus and herpes simplex virus infections in Greenland and Denmark: a population-based study. *American Journal of Epidemiology*, **131**, 1980, p 669.

56. Rosenberg, M.J. *et al.* Effect of the contraceptive sponge on chlamydial infection, gonorrhoea and candidiasis. *Journal of the American Medical Association*, **257**, 1987, pp 2308–12.

57. Fleissig A, Unintended pregnancy and the use of contraception: changes from 1984 to 1989. *British Medical Journal,* **302**, 1991, p 147.

58. Bromham, D. R. *et al.* Knowledge and use of secondary contraception among patients requesting termination of pregnancy. *British Medical Journal*, **306**, 1993, pp 556–7.

59. Duncan, G. *et al.* Termination of pregnancy, lessons for prevention. *British Journal of Family Planning*, **15**, 1990, pp 112–17.

60. *Emergency Contraception Campaign: an evaluation.* London: HEA, 1997.

61. George, J. *et al.* Women's knowledge of emergency contraception. *British Journal of General Practice*, **44**, 1994, pp 451–4.

62. Thomas, P. *Awareness and availability of emergency contraception in a South Wales valley. Raising awareness about emergency contraception : report of a conference organised by Health Promotion Wales, 2 November 1993.* Health Promotion Wales, 1994.

63. Graham, A. *et al.* Teenagers' knowledge of emergency contraception: questionnaire survey in south-east Scotland. *British Medical Journal*, **312**, 1996, pp 1567–9.

64. Lumb, J. Postcoital contraception. *Pharmaceutical Journal,* **253**, 1994, pp 540–1.

65. Walsh, J. Policies and practices in postcoital contraceptive provision: a survey of general practitioners and hospital accident and emergency departments. *British Journal of Family Planning,* **20**, 1995, pp 121–5.

66. Walsh, J. Family planning provision within genitourinary medicine clinics: a quiet revolution. *British Journal of Family Planning,* **22**, 1996, pp 27–30.

67. Family Planning Association. *Use of family planning services in the United Kingdom*. Factsheet 1B. London: FPA, 1996.

68. Pearson, V. A. H. *et al.* Family planning services in Devon, UK: awareness, experience and attitudes of pregnant teenagers. *British Journal of Family Planning,* **21**, 1995, pp 45–9.

69. Department of Health. *Health and personal social services: statistics for England*. HMSO, 1995.

70. Snowden, R. *Consumer choices in family planning*. FPA, 1985.

71. Bromham, D. R. and Cartmill, R. S. V. Are current sources of contraceptive advice adequate to meet the changes in contraceptive practice? A study of patients requesting termination of pregnancy. *British Journal of Family Planning,* **19**, 1993, pp 170–83.

Abortion

1. Office of National Statistics. *Birth Statistics 1994*. Series FM1, No. 23. HMSO, 1996.

2. Office for National Statistics. *Legal Abortions 1995*. Series AB 96/6. ONS, 1996.

3. Office for National Statistics. *Legal Abortions 1995*. Series AB 96/5. ONS, 1996.

4. Botting, B. Trends in abortion. *Population Trends*, **64**, 1991, pp 19–29.

5. Ashton, J. R. Trends in induced abortion in England and Wales. *British Medical Journal*, **287**, 1983, pp 1001–2.

6. Social and Community Planning Research. *British social attitudes: cumulative resource book*. SCPR, 1992.

7. Royal College of Obstetricians and Gynaecologists. *Report of the RCOG Working Party on Unplanned Pregnancy*. London: RCOG, 1991.

8. Duncan, G. *et al.* Termination of pregnancy: lessons for prevention. *British Journal of Family Planning,* **15**, 1990, pp 112–17.

9. Office of Population Censuses and Surveys/Office of National Statistics. *Legal abortions 1992, 1993, 1994.* Series AB, Nos 19/20/21. HMSO, 1994 and 1995.

10. Smith, T. Influence of socio-economic factors on attaining targets for reducing teenage pregnancies. *British Medical Journal,* **306**, 1993, pp 1232–5.

11. Bruce, N. *Reducing unplanned pregnancy – an investigation of abortion in Camden and Islington.* Hampstead Health Authority, 1992.

12. Office of Population Censuses and Surveys. *County Monitors.* Series CEN 91 CM 1– CEN 91 CM 54. OPCS, 1992.

13. David, H. P. Abortion in Europe, 1920–91: a public health perspective. *Studies in Family Planning,* **23** (1), 1992, pp 1–22.

14. Henshaw, S. Induced abortion: a world review. *Family Planning Perspectives,* **22** (2), 1990, pp 76–89.

15. Singh, S. and Henshaw, S. Socio-cultural and political aspects of abortion from an anthropological perspective. Paper presented at IUSSP seminar, Trivandrum, India, 1996.

16. Brook Advisory Centres. *Directory of Birth Control Services for Young People.* Brook Advisory Centres, 1994.

17. Scally, G. and Hadley, A. Accessibility of sexual health services for young people: survey of clinics in a region. *Journal of Management in Medicine,* **9**, 1995, pp 51–2.

18. Pearson, V. A. H. *et al.* Teenage pregnancy: a comparative study of teenagers choosing termination of pregnancy or antenatal care. *Journal of the Royal Society of Medicine,* **88**, 1995, pp 384–8.

19. *Report of the Royal Commission on National Health Service.* Cmnd 7615. HMSO, 1979.

20. Allen, I. *Counselling services for sterilisation, vasectomy and termination of pregnancy.* Policy Studies Institute, 1985.

21. Clarke. L. *et al.* The views and experiences of women having NHS and private treatment: Camden abortion study. *British Pregnancy Advisory Service,* 1983.

22. Pro-choice Alliance/ Pregnancy Advisory Service. *Survey of abortion patients.* Pro-choice Alliance, 1993.

23. Hartnell, V. H. Medical termination of pregnancy and the future provision of termination services. *British Journal of Family Planning,* **19**, 1993, pp 143–4.

24. Tietze, C. and Henshaw S. K. *Induced abortion: a world review.* New York: Alan Guttmacher Institute, 1986.

25. Baulecu, E. RU486 as an anti-progestogen steroid. *Journal of the American Medical Association,* **262**, 1983, pp 1808–14.

26. Silvestre, L. The French experience. In: *The abortion pill – widening the choice for women.* London: Birth Control Trust, 1990.

27. Cameron, I. T. and Baird, D. T. Early pregnancy termination – a comparison between vacuum aspiration and medical abortion using prostaglandin or the anti-progestogen RU486. *British Journal of Obstetrics and Gynaecology,* **96**, 1988, pp 271–6.

28. Saha, A. Savage, W. and George, J. *The Tower Hamlets Daycare Abortion Service Study.* Doctors for a Woman's Choice on Abortion, 1992.

29. Glasier, A. The establishment of a centralised referral service leads to earlier abortion. *Health Bulletin,* **49** (5), 1991, pp 254–9.

AIDS and HIV

1. Gunson, H. H. and Rawlinson, V. I. Screening of blood donations for HIV-1 antibody 1985-1991. *Communicable Disease Report,* **1**, Review 13, 1991, pp R144–R146.

2. Keet, I. P .M. *et al.* Oro-genital sex and the transmission of HIV among homosexual men. *AIDS,* **6** (2), 1992, pp 223–6.

3. WHO. The current global situation of AIDS, 30 June 1996.

4. UNAIDS: HIV/AIDS figures and trends mid-1996 estimates, June 1996.

5. UN AIDS and WHO: the HIV/AIDS situation in mid-1996 Global and regional highlights, 1996.

6. European centre for the Epidemiological Monitoring of AIDS. *AIDS Surveillance in Europe.* Quarterly Report No. 51, 1996.

7. PHLS. CDSC. The surveillance of HIV-1 infection and AIDS in England and Wales. *Communicable Disease Report,* **1** (5), 1991, R51-R56.

8. PHLS CDSC. The incidence and prevalence of AIDS and prevalence of other severe HIV disease in England and Wales for 1995 to 1999: projections (using data to end of 1994). Report of an Expert Advisory Group (Chairman: Professor N. E. Day) convened by the Director of the Public Health Laboratory Service on behalf of the Chief Medical Officer. *Communicable Disease Report,* **6**, Review 1, 5 January 1996.

9. PHLS AIDS Centre. CDSC. Unlinked anonymous HIV prevalence monitoring in England and Wales: 1990–1994. Report from Unlinked HIV Surveys Steering Group. Department of Health, 1995.

10. PHLS AIDS Centre. CDSC and Scottish Centre for Infection and Environmental Health. Unpublished quarterly surveillance tables, No. 32, June 1996.

11. PHLS. CDSC. AIDS and HIV infection in the United Kingdom: monthly report. *Communicable Disease Report*, **6** (16), 1996, pp 141–4.

12. Home Office. *Statistical Bulletin,* May 1993.

13. Brenner, H. *et al. AIDS among drug users in Europe.* Copenhagen: WHO, 1991.

14. Department of Health and the Welsh Office. *Short-term prediction of HIV infection and AIDS in England and Wales: Report of a Working Group.* London: HMSO, 1988.

15. PHLS CDSC. Acquired immune deficiency syndrome in England and Wales to end 1993: projections using data to end September 1989. Report of a Working Group convened by the Director of the Public Health Laboratory Service. *Communicable Disease Report.* January 1990.

16. PHLS CDSC. The incidence and prevalence of AIDS and other severe HIV disease in England and Wales for 1992–1997: projections using data to the end of June 1992. Report of an expert working group (Chairman: Professor N.E. Day) convened by the Director of the Public Health Laboratory Service on behalf of the Chief Medical Officers. *Communicable Disease Report*, **3**, Supplement, 1 June 1993.

17. Wellings, K., Field, J. *et al. Sexual behaviour in Britain: the national survey of sexual attitudes and lifestyles.* Penguin Books, 1994.

18. Knox, E. G. *et al. Sexual behaviour and AIDS in Britain.* HMSO, 1993.

19. Scottish Centre for Infection and Environmental Health. *AIDS and severe HIV-related disease in Scotland: predictions to the end of 1999.* SCIEH, Glasgow, 1995.

20. FitzSimons D. *et al.* (eds) *The economic and social impact of AIDS in Europe.* London: National AIDS Trust, 1995.

21. House of Commons, Health Committee, first report. Session 1994/95. *Priority setting in the NHS: purchasing.* Volume 1: Report together with Annexes and Proceedings of the Committee. London: HMSO, 1995.

22. Editorial. *Economist*, 29 June1996.

23. Aldous, J. *et al.* Impact of HIV infection on mortality in young men in a London health authority. *British Medical Journal*, **305**, 1992, pp 219–21.

24. Gray, A. M. *Economic aspects of AIDS and HIV infection in the UK.* London School of Hygiene and Tropical Medicine, 1991.

25. Department of Health. Personal communication.

26. Brown, P. Has the AIDS research epidemic spread too far? *New Scientist*, 15 May 1993, pp 12–15.

27. Keynote Report. *Contraceptives.* London: Keynote, 1993.

28. Health Education Authority. *AIDS Strategic Monitor* (January 1990 – February 1991) survey carried out by BMRB on behalf of the HEA. London: HEA, 1994.

29. Health Education Authority. *Communications Monitor.* (AIDS Module). Carried out by BMRB on behalf of the HEA. October 1993. Unpublished.

30. Health Education Authority. AIDS Awareness (February/March 1996) carried out by BMRB on behalf of the HEA. Unpublished, 1996.

31. Health Education Authority. *Health and lifestyle survey: a survey of the UK population*, Part 1. Carried out by MORI on behalf of the HEA, 1995.

Sexually transmitted diseases other than HIV infection

1. Washington, A. E., Cates, W. Jr. and Wasserheit, J. N. Preventing pelvic inflammatory disease. *Journal of the American Medical Association*, **266**, 1991, pp 2574–80

2. Catchpole, M. Sexually transmitted diseases in England and Wales 1981–1991. *Communicable Disease Report*, No.1, 1992, R1–R6.

3. Office of Health Economics. *OHE Compendium of Health Statistics.* London: OHE, 1995.

4. Plummer, F. A. *et al.* Co-factors in the male/female transmission of Human Immunodeficiency Virus 1. *Journal of Infectious Disease*, **163**, 1991, pp 233–9.

5. Quinn, T. C. Global burden of the HIV pandemic. *Lancet*, **347** (9020), 1996, pp 99–106.

6. Department of Health. Statistical Bulletin 1996/4. *Sexually transmitted diseases, England, 1995: new cases seen at NHS Genito-Urinary Medicine Clinics.*

7. British Federation Against Sexually Transmitted Diseases. Secretary's Report, 1996. Unpublished.

8. Whatley, J., Thin, N. *et al.* Problems of adolescent sexuality. *Journal of the Royal Society of Medicine*, **82**, 1989, pp 732–4.

9. PHLS CDSC. Sexually transmitted diseases quarterly report: gonorrhoea in England and Wales. *Communicable Disease Report,* **6** (13), 1996, pp 110–11.

10. Carnes, C., Weller, I. V. D. *et al.* Prevalence of antibodies to human immunodeficiency virus, gonorrhoea rates and changed sexual behaviour in homosexual men in London. *Lancet*, **i**, (8534),1987, pp 656–8.

11. Hunt, A. J. *et al.* (Project SIGMA) Changes in sexual behaviour in a large cohort of homosexual men in England and Wales, 1988-9. *British Medical Journal*, **302**, 1991, pp 505–6.

12. Allen, I. and Hogg, D. *Work roles and responsibilities in genitourinary medicine clinics*. Policy Studies Institute, 1993.

13. Evans, B. G. *et al.* Sexually transmitted diseases and HIV-1 infection among homosexual men in England and Wales. *British Medical Journal*, **306**, 1993, pp 426–8.

14. Riley, V. C. Resurgent gonorrhoea in homosexual men. *Lancet*, **337**, 1991, p 183.

15. French, P. D. *et al.* Preventing the spread of HIV infection. *British Medical Journal*, **302**, 1991, p 962.

16. Whitaker, L. and Renton, A. A theoretical problem of interpreting the recently reported increase in homosexual gonorrhoea. *European Journal of Epidemiology*, **8**, 1992, pp 187–91.

17. Mabey, D. Editorial comment on papers of outstanding interest (epidemiology). *Current AIDS Literature*, **6** (5), 1993, pp 183–4.

18. Health Education Authority. *AIDS Awareness 2 (combined)* (February/March 1996) Carried out by BMRB on behalf of the HEA. London: HEA, 1996. Unpublished.

19. Department of Health. *The health of the nation: a strategy for health in England*. Cm 1986. HMSO, 1992.

20. Department of Health. *GUM clinic returns 1990*. (Annual and December quarter figures). Summary information from form KC60. Department of Health, 1991.

21. Van der Hoek, J. A. R. *et al.* Increase in unsafe homosexual behaviour. *Lancet*, **336**, 1990, pp 179–80.

22. Singaratnam, A. E. *et al.* Preventing the spread of HIV infection. *British Medical Journal*, **302**, 1991, p 469.

23. Beck, E. J. *et al.* Case-control study of sexually transmitted diseases as cofactors for HIV-1 transmission. *International Journal of STD and AIDS*, **7**, 1997, pp 34–8.

24. Renton, A. M. and Whitaker, L. *Using STD occurrence to monitor AIDS prevention*. Report for the EC concerted action 'Assessment of AIDS/HIV preventive strategies'. London: St Mary's Hospital Medical School, 1992.

25. Whoolley, D. P. *et al.* Fear of HIV infection and reduction in heterosexual gonorrhoea. *British Medical Journal*, **296**, 1988, p 1199.

26. Gellan, M. C. A. and Ison, C. A. Declining incidence of gonorrhoea in London: A response to fear of AIDS? *Lancet*, **ii**, 1986, p 920.

27. PHLS/CDSC. *Unlinked anonymous HIV prevalence monitoring in England and Wales*: 1990–1994. Report from the unlinked HIV surveys steering group. Department of Health, 1995.

28. Hudson, C. P. Concurrent partnerships could cause AIDS epidemic. *International Journal of STD and AIDS*, **4**, 1993, pp 249-53

29. Tomlinson, D. R. *et al.* Does rectal gonorrhoea reflect unsafe sex? *Lancet*, **337**, 1991, p 501.

30. Waight, P. A. and Miller E. Incidence of HIV infection among homosexual men. *British Medical Journal*, **303**, 1991, p 311.

Sex education in schools

1. Family Planning Association. *Children who have children*. FPA, 1993.

2. Brook Advisory Centres. *Annual Report 1991–92*. London: Brook Advisory Centres, 1992.

3. Allen. I. *Family planning and pregnancy counselling projects for young people*, London: Policy Studies Institute, 1991.

4. World Health Organization. *School health education to prevent AIDS and sexually transmitted diseases*. WHO AIDS Series 10. Geneva: WHO, 1992.

5. Department of Health. *The health of the nation: a strategy for health in England*. Cm 1986. London: HMSO, 1992.

6. Kirby, D. *et al.* School-based programmes to reduce sexual risk behaviours: a review of effectiveness. *Public Health Reports* (US), **109**, 1994, pp 339–60.

7. Wellings, K. *et al.* Provision of sex education and early sexual experience: the relation examined. *British Medical Journal*, **311**, 1995, pp 417–20.

8. Department for Education. *Statistics of Education: Schools*. Department for Education, 1992.

9. Department for Education. *Education Act 1993: Sex Education in Schools*. Circular No. 5/94.

10. National Curriculum Council. *Curriculum Guidance 5: Health Education*. NCC, 1990.

11. School Curriculum and Assessment Authority. *Science in the National Curriculum*. London: HMSO, 1994.

12. Health Education Authority. *Health education in schools – a survey of head teachers and health co-ordinators*. Carried out by MORI on behalf of the HEA in 1989. London: HEA, 1989.

13. Thomson, R. and Scott, L. *An enquiry into sex education.* Report of a survey into local education authority support and monitoring of school education, compiled on behalf of the Sex Education Forum. London: Sex Education Forum, 1992.

14. Aggleton, P. and Toft, M. *Young people, sexual health and HIV/AIDS promotion.* A discussion paper prepared for the Health Education Authority. London: HEA, 1991. Unpublished.

15. Massey, D. E. School sex education: knitting without a pattern? *Health Education Journal,* **49** (3), 1990, pp 134–42.

16. Health Education Authority. *A survey of health education policies in schools.* Carried out by NFER on behalf of the HEA. London: HEA, 1993.

17. Health Education Authority. *Today's young adults: 16–19-year-olds look at diet, alcohol, smoking, drugs and sexual behaviour.* London: HEA, 1992.

18. Health Education Authority. *Young people and health: the health behaviour of school aged children.* London: HEA, 1997.

19. National AIDS Trust. *Living for tomorrow.* London: NAT, 1991.

20. Mellanby, A. *et al.* Teenagers and the risks of sexually transmitted diseases: a need for the provision balanced information. *Genitourinary Medicine,* **68**, 1992, pp 241–4.

21. HEA. *Health and lifestyles: a survey of the UK population,* Part 1. Conducted by MORI on behalf of the Health Education Authority. London: HEA, 1995.

22. HEA and National Foundation for Educational Research in England and Wales. *Parents, schools and sex education – a compelling case for partnership.* Summary of the main report conducted for the Health Education Authority. London: HEA, 1994.

Appendix 1

1. Barre-Sinoussi, F. *et al.* Isolation of T-lymphotropic retrovirus from a patient at risk for acquired immune deficiency syndrome (AIDS). *Science,* **220**, 1983, pp 868–71.

2. Popovic, M. *et al.* Detection, isolation and continuous production of cytopathic retroviruses (HTLV-III) from patients with AIDS and pre-AIDS. *Science,* **224**, 1984, p 497.

3. Gallo, R.C. *et al.* Frequent detection and isolation of cytopathic retroviruses (HTLV-III) from patients with AIDS and at risk for AIDS. *Science,* **224**, 1984, pp 500–3.

4. Schupbach, J. *et al.* Serological analysis of a subgroup of human T-lymphotropic retroviruses (HTLV-III) associated with AIDS. *Science,* **224**, 1984, p 503.

5. Sarngadharan, M.G. *et al.* Antibodies reactive with human T-lymphotropic retroviruses (HTLV-III) in the serum of patients with AIDS. *Science,* **224**, 1991, p 506.

6. Rowland-Jones, S. *et al.* HIV-specific cytotoxic T-cells in HIV-exposed but uninfected Gambian women. *Nature Medicine,* **1** (1), 1995, pp 59-64.

7. Quinn, T. C. Global burden of the HIV pandemic, *Lancet,* **348**, 1996 (13 July), pp 99–106.

8. Osborn, J. E. HIV: the more things change, the more they stay the same, *Nature Medicine,* **1** (10), 1995, pp 991–3.

9. Gottlieb, M. S. *et al.* Pneumocystis carinii pneumonia and mucosal candidiasis in previously healthy homosexual men: evidence of a new acquired cellular immunodeficiency. *New England Journal of Medicine,* **305**, 1981, p 1425.

10. Masur, H. An outbreak of community-acquired pneumocystis carinii pneumonia: initial manifestation of cellular immune dysfunction. *New England Journal of Medicine,* **305**, 1981, p 1431.

11. Seigal, F. P. Severe acquired immunodeficiency in male homosexuals, manifested by chronic perianal ulcerative herpes simplex lesions. *New England Journal of Medicine,* **305**, 1981, p 1439.

12. PHLS CDSC. Case definitions for AIDS – Europe and the United States part company. *Communicable Disease Report,* **3** (4), 1993, p 1.

13. Rutherford, G. W. *et al.* Course of HIV-1 infection in a cohort of homosexual and bisexual men: an 11 year follow up study. *British Medical Journal,* **301**, 1990, p 1183.

14. Pantaleo, G. and Fauci, A. S. New concepts in the immunopathogenesis of HIV infection. *Annual Review of Immunology,* **13**, 1995, pp 487–512.

15. Whitmore-Overton, S. E. *et al.* Improved survival from diagnosis of AIDS in adult cases in the United Kingdom and bias due to reporting delays. *AIDS,* **7** (3), 1993, pp 415–20.

Appendix 3

1. PHLS AIDS Centre. The surveillance of HIV-1 infection and AIDS in England and Wales. *Communicable Disease Report,* **1** (5), 1991, R51–R56.

2. Evans, B.G. *et al.* Surveillance of HIV infection and AIDS in the UK: an overview from the PHLS AIDS Centre. *PHLS Microbiology Digest,* **10** (3), 1993, pp 141–3.

10M/059/7